C000263559

PENIS GENIUS

Jordan LaRousse & Samantha Sade

QUIVER

Brimming with creative inspiration, how-to projects, and useful information to enrich your everyday life, Quarto Knows is a favorite destination for those pursuing their interests and passions. Visit our site and dig deeper with our books into your area of interest: Quarto Creates, Quarto Cooks, Quarto Homes, Quarto Lives, Quarto Drives, Quarto Explores, Quarto Gifts, or Quarto Kids.

Inspiring | Educating | Creating | Entertaining

First Published in 2018 by Fair Winds Press, an imprint of The Quarto Group,
100 Cummings Center, Suite 265-D, Beverly, MA 01915, USA.
T (978) 282-9590 F (978) 283-2742 QuartoKnows.com

Fair Winds Press titles are also available at discount for retail, wholesale, promotional, and bulk purchase. For details, contact the Special Sales Manager by email at specialsales@quarto.com or by mail at The Quarto Group, Attn: Special Sales Manager, 401 Second Avenue North, Suite 310, Minneapolis, MN 55401, USA.

The Publisher maintains the records relating to images in this book required by 18 USC 2257. Records are located at The Quarto Group, 100 Cummings Center, Suite 265-D, Beverly, MA 01915, USA.

The content for this book originally appeared in *Penis Genius* (Quiver 2011) by Jordan LaRousse and Samantha Sade.

22 21 20 19 18   3 4 5

ISBN: 978-1-59233-795-8

Digital edition published in 2018

Cover design/illustration by www.gordonbeveridge.com
Book layout by Sporto
Photography by Holly Randall

Printed and bound in Hong Kong

ODE TO THE PENIS

Life without penis would be a droopy, dreary place. There would be no dick jokes, erections, cock rings, or Caverject injections; there would be no place to hang your condom, no baby batter, and no big hard-ons. We wish to examine the cock's ins and outs, from its helmetlike head to the way it spouts. We say hooray for the penis in all of its glory, whether the size of a shrimp or eleven full stories.

CONTENTS

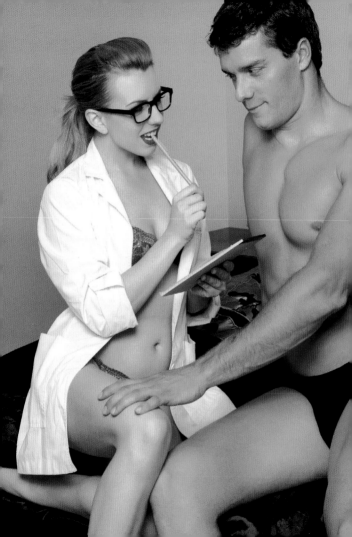

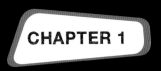

CHAPTER 1

PENIS ANATOMY: A PLEASURE ROAD MAP

You may have seen a detailed illustration
of penis anatomy at your doctor's office,
but this lesson is unlike any your M.D.
would ever give you. From corona to
shaft, from frenulum to scrotum, we'll
give you a step-by-step road map of his
pleasure stick, and along the way we'll let
you know which parts are most
responsive to sexual stimulation and how
to expertly handle them. We'll also let you
know which areas to be careful around.
(The meatus, for example, is extremely
sensitive to alcohol; this is one case where
meat and wine don't mix!)

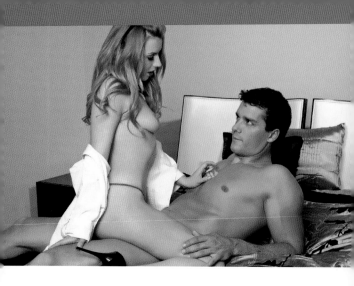

PENIS SHAFT

Where to Find It

The penis shaft is that shape-shifting pillar of flesh that sometimes (or quite often when in your sexy presence) juts out from between his legs. When flaccid (due to cold temperatures, anxiety, mundane activities, and surprise visits from your mother), it does a lot less jutting and hangs freely between his legs. It might appear shriveled and loose, or completely bundled up like a turtle in its shell.

Its Purpose

Without a shaft, there would be nothing to erect for his erection. The shaft contains three columns of spongy erectile tissue; two are called *corpora cavernosa*, and the third, which wraps around the urethra, is the *corpora spongiosum*. The tissue is interlaced by a network of arteries that, when aroused, fill up with blood, creating a sight that most women are very familiar with: the raging hard-on. After ejaculation, dorsal veins drain the blood out of his penis (and hopefully send it back to his brain).

Indications/Contraindications

As the largest area of his penis, his shaft offers a ton of fun to be had. Wrap your hands around it and stroke, wrap your lips around it and lick and suck, wrap your breasts around it and titty-fuck, and of course wrap your legs around it and ride. Or make fast little licks on the underside of the shaft—sideways, instead of up and down.

The base of the shaft begins inside his body, underneath the testicles. You can access this part of his shaft by pressing your forefinger or hand, lengthwise, to the center of his scrotum. Use slow, careful pressure to separate the testicles. Gently rub back and forth until you get to the base of the scrotum, where you will indirectly make contact with the hidden bottom of his shaft. If he likes it, continue the massage.

Much like the interior of your vaginal canal (as opposed to your labia and clitoris), the shaft of your man's penis is very responsive to pressure. Stimulating the head of his cock and surrounding areas with your tongue while keeping a firm or pulsating grip on his shaft may be just what the doctor ordered.

It's hard to go wrong with the shaft, but unless your guy is into penile pain, don't bite, don't pull on it like a tug rope, and *please* don't give him any Indian rug burns.

GLANS PENIS

Where to Find It

Glans penis is the scientific word for his little head (as opposed to his big head, which is where he presumably keeps his brain). It's the helmet that sits atop the shaft, and it houses a great number of nerve endings.

Its Purpose

Among other unusual attributes—like fully opposable thumbs, an inexplicable love for televised sports, and (compared to other primates) relatively hair-free skin—human males are the only species who have a little head below their belts. This has caused scientists to wonder about the evolutionary purpose of this bulbous addition to his shaft. The unique mushroom shape, aside from being integral to your pleasure, has been postulated to serve an important evolutionary purpose that increases a man's potential for creating offspring.

Indications/Contraindications

Second only to the frenulum, 26 percent of our male survey takers reported that stimulation of the penis head was the most stimulating. Because of the high concentration of nerve endings and the consequent pleasure principle, the glans penis has been compared to the highly sensitive clitoris. In fact, the two develop from the same tissue in the womb. Now that you can empathize with this sensitive spot, you understand the importance of lavishing it with attention. Try licking it like an ice cream cone and use generous flicks of your tongue. Suck it like a lollipop, or treat it like a pleasurable frosting spatula by taking his shaft in your hand and using the glans to spread the juices of your slick vaginal lips or to stimulate your clit.

Use common sense. Just as you wouldn't want him to rub your clit raw, treat him the same by keeping your touch slippery and soft.

CORONA

Where to Find It

No, we're not talking about a refreshing bottle of beer garnished with a slice of lime. Corona is Spanish for *crown*, and it describes that little ridge of flesh that separates the head of his cock from the shaft.

Its Purpose

Some scientists conjecture that the corona (or coronal ridge), aside from making his penis look like royalty, also serves as a semen displacement device. In 2003, a team of psychologists from the State University of New York hypothesized that the corona is shaped specifically so that it can scrape other men's semen out of a woman's vaginal canal, by way of vigorous thrusting. The purpose is to eliminate genetic competition.

To test this hypothesis, the team used a fake pussy, of the type found at your local sex store, and three dildos, one with a large coronal ridge, another with a smaller ridge, and a third without any ridge at all. They filled the fake vagina with the semen-alternative (flour and water) and then, using each phallus in turn, recreated a thrusting motion, similar to the one your guy treats you to during a hot round of coitus. The result? Both dildos with the coronal ridges displaced 91 percent of the semen, while the headless toy only displaced 35 percent of the gunk. They also found that the deeper the thrust, the more semen was displaced.

Think about the possible implications of this study! It could indicate that men have evolved to compete for reproduction rights with women who are, by nature, not monogamous. This could support the idea that humans are not wired for monogamy at all. (Oh behave, you little trollops!)

Indications/Contraindications

As a part of his glans, the flesh around the corona is very sensitive to pleasure. With sensitivity to pleasure comes sensitivity to pain. Handle with care.

FRENULUM

Where to Find It

Everyone has several frenula on their body; find one of yours by licking along the upper front side of your gums where they meet the inside of your upper lip. Feel that taught membrane? That is a frenulum. Your guy just so happens to have one on the underside of his penis where the glans and shaft connect.

Its Purpose

On uncircumcised men, the frenulum helps the foreskin slide back and forth over the glans. On circumcised men, this little piece of his penis has nothing to support or restrain, so it serves more as a pleasure spot than anything else.

Indications/Contraindications

In our survey, 41 percent of men said their frenulum is the most sensitive spot on their cocks. Lightly caress and lick this area during sex play. Try massaging the area with your thumb using soft, circular motions, while caressing his glans with the rest of your fingers. If you are eager for your guy to ejaculate, a rhythmic stroking of this particular spot could do the trick.

Some uncircumcised men may have a condition called *frenulum breve*, which is a shortened frenulum. For these guys, it's difficult for the foreskin to pull back completely from the glans, and it can cause painful sex or even little tears in the sensitive flesh. Men with this condition are often told that the only solution is circumcision. However, there is another, less invasive procedure called frenuloplasty, a ten-minute outpatient method that loosens the frenulum so that the foreskin can properly retract.

FORESKIN

Where to Find It

In the United States, it may be difficult to find the foreskin. (We are a foreskin-challenged nation!) According to the U.S. Department of Health and Human Services, currently 60 percent of American males had their foreskins removed via circumcision in infancy. However, if you encounter an intact penis, you'll notice the foreskin resembles a cozy little sleeping bag that covers the head of his penis when it's flaccid. When erect, the glans comes out from its shell, and the foreskin appears more like a bunched up sock just beneath the head. Foreskin is elastic and mobile, and can be a source of great pleasure.

Its Purpose

The foreskin (also known as the prepuce) protects his glans from irritation and chafing, creates natural lubrication during masturbation and sex, facilitates penetration during sex (reducing friction and eliminating the need to "force" it in), and contains a high density of nerve endings that enhance his pleasure.

Indications/Contraindications

When giving a hand job or blow job, don't neglect this erogenous zone. Try moving the elastic flesh of the foreskin up and down over his glans. The area just inside the tip of his foreskin is particularly sensitive to pleasure—try gently massaging the inside, or flick your tongue under the skin and around the "lips" of the foreskin (where it opens for the glans).

The biggest concern with intact men is cleanliness. Small glands beneath the foreskin produce a cheesy, stinky substance called smegma. To avoid irritation and infection, it's important for men to keep their parts clean and tidy and not allow the substance to build up. Nothing can ruin a blow job faster than the overpowering scent of Camembert in his shorts.

MEATUS

Where to Find It
The meatus is the little slit at the top of his glans.

Its Purpose
No, the meatus isn't the eye of the one-eyed wonder worm! It's the opening of the urethra, where both urine and semen exit the penis.

Indications/Contraindications
Using either a lubricated palm or finger, or your tongue, you can gently massage or lick the opening. Sensitive mucous membranes around the opening can be susceptible to pleasure if touched wetly and lightly.

These sensitive mucous membranes can be easily irritated. A lot of men would prefer you not to tread too closely to this spot, so be careful. If your guy is open to a little meatus stimulation, never use a dry hand around this area because it can cause the slit to uncomfortably pull open and you can even accidentally scrape him.

It's best not to introduce irritating substances such as alcohol or hot chili peppers to the meatus, which can sting when they come in contact with that tiny opening, just like rubbing alcohol stings when you rub it on a cut. Other spicy or acidic foods may have the same effect. So, unless your guy is into pain, try a cool glass of water instead.

Note that sexually transmitted infections can be passed through this opening. Use condoms, and keep your mouth away if you have sores or cuts.

SCROTUM

Where to Find It
The scrotum is that oft-ignored sack of flesh containing his testicles that hangs below your man's penis.

Its Purpose
The main function is to keep the testicles at the optimum temperature for generating sperm. While the rest of the body is comfortable at 98.6°F (37°C), the testes prefer a cooler temperature of 93°F (34°C), keeping the little swimmers at the ready for action. When things get a little too cold for comfort outside, the scrotum wrinkles and tightens, hugging the testicles close to the body for added warmth.

Indications/Contraindications
Although it may not look as beautiful as your guy's penis, the scrotum is a powerhouse of pleasure. Try gently tugging down on his sack as you give him a blow job. During a hand job, try very gently sucking first one testicle and then the other into your mouth. To give him a real sensory treat, lick or caress the line that runs down the center of his scrotum. This little treasure trail is called the scrotal raphe, pronounced *RAY-fee*.

Don't be too rough with his family jewels. Since the scrotum contains the very sensitive testes, avoid jabbing, hitting, or knocking these guys together. For men, getting hit in the nuts is one of the most painful things to endure. Take heart and spare him the pain so he can trust you with his fun little playthings.

Once you have your guy's penis mapped out, it's time for a sexy expedition. Travel, explore, and enjoy his unique hot spots. He'll be dubbing you a penis genius before you know it!

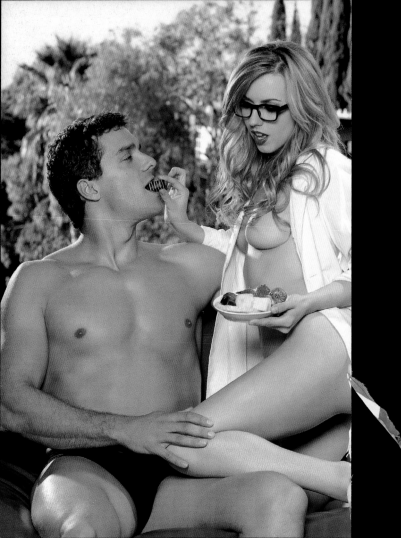

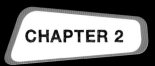

CHAPTER 2

HIS SPECIAL SAUCE: ALL THE FLAVORS OF HIS PUDDING

Ejaculation is the final show in a man's typical sexual encounter. From the money-shot so often and openly displayed in porn, to his final grunts and spasms during coitus, the eruption of semen can be compared to the fireworks finale at a New Year's Eve party. As such, the mysterious substance lends itself to a variety of questions, concerns, and lore.

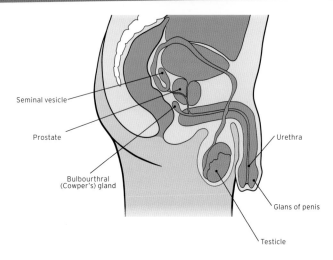

Seminal vesicle

Prostate

Bulbourthral
(Cowper's) gland

Urethra

Glans of penis

Testicle

For starters, let's get the facts straight about the difference between semen and sperm. Semen is the sticky fluid that erupts from your guy's penis when you bring him to orgasm. Usually, he'll shoot about a teaspoon of the stuff for each ejaculation. The seminal fluid carries the little baby makers known as spermatozoa, or sperm. There are approximately 200 million to 500 million sperm in each ejaculation, but they are so tiny that they only make up about 1 percent of the total concoction.

There are a lot of cooks in the semen kitchen. The testicles are responsible for producing the actual sperm, but only about 5 percent of the total seminal fluid. The rest of the brew is produced by various glands in your guy's body. The seminal vesicles, for example, produce the seminal plasma—think of this as the thickening base ingredient in your man's soup—which makes up about 45 percent to 80 percent of the total fluid. The prostate gland contributes 15 percent to 30 percent of semen's volume in the form of prostate fluid, which we like to think of as a flavorful preservative. This milky, alkaline fluid neutralizes the acidity in a woman's vagina and uterus, helping to protect the sperm as they make the arduous trek toward the egg. Other glands providing smaller amounts of seasoning to the tasty concoction include the bulbourethral (Cowper's) and urethral glands.

PRESENTATION OF THE SEMEN SOUP

Now that we have a basic understanding of the recipe for ejaculate, let's talk about its presentation. The delivery of semen is a pointedly interactive experience for both parties, and because of this, you and your lover may have an array of questions about its color, consistency, taste, potency, and even the amount that comes out.

Why Is Some Cum Watery While Other Spooge Is Creamy?

If real life were like the porn industry, all men would shoot spurt after spurt of creamy, milky white semen. In reality, semen varies in color, quantity, and consistency from man to man and even from orgasm to orgasm. The variation is due to a number of factors, including how much water your man has been drinking (more water can help produce more semen) and how many times he's ejaculated in a specific time span (if he's not given time to build up his reserves, the amount of cum will decrease with each shot). It's normal for semen to be white, yellowish, or even grey in color. Note: Pink semen may indicate the presence of blood, and if it persists, he should seek medical attention.

If your guy doesn't ejaculate at all when he orgasms, he's likely experiencing retrograde ejaculation, where the semen goes backward in his urethra down to the bladder instead of shooting out the meatus. Retrograde ejaculation is rare and, in and of itself, is not a major health concern unless you're trying to get pregnant. However, retrograde ejaculation can be a side effect of certain high blood pressure and mood-altering medications, surgery, or diabetes, in which cases your man should consult with his physician to manage the cause.

Is It Possible to Increase the Volume of Ejaculate?

Many men seem to be concerned with producing a nice, healthy helping of baby batter, whether or not they're actually trying to make a baby. Some men may correlate a large helping to impressive sexual prowess. There is a small amount of biology behind the desire for an increased volume of semen. A larger amount means more sperm (and thus a greater chance of impregnation), as well as more or stronger muscle contractions required to spurt the stuff out (and thus more pleasurable orgasms).

Unfortunately, there's not a lot of hard science to inform us on how to increase seminal volume. Some sex experts recommend amino acids such as L-arginine and L-lysine, zinc, as well as Horny Goat Weed plant. Increasing fluids is another suggestion. And abstaining from coming for a day or two (rather than an hour or two) will ensure optimum semen levels.

How Far Should Semen Shoot?

When unhindered, the first contraction of a male ejaculation can propel his semen one to two feet (0.3 to 0.6 meters). However, some

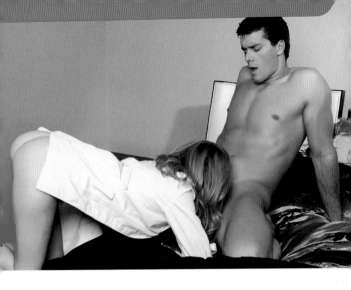

men may experience only a small dribble of ejaculate upon orgasm. Both scenarios are normal, and neither are cause for concern. Internet lore reports that a man named Horst Schultz achieved an ejaculation that shot 18 feet, 9 inches at 42.7 miles per hour (about 5.7 meters at 68.7 km/hour). Even if this is possible, unless your guy is a secret agent and needs to be able to use his penis as a weapon, what's the point? During sex, his cock is typically inside some orifice of your body or contained in a condom, and the actual distance he can ejaculate is null.

What Semens to Be the Problem?

It's all naughty fun and games until someone gets semen in the eye. If this happens to you, don't panic! The stuff stings about as much as a dollop of shampoo and it's as easily treated. Simply rinse your eye out with cool water.

There is a small chance that you can contract an STI from semen-to-eye contact (especially diseases such as chlamydia and gonorrhea), so watch for any rashes or sores that may develop, especially if you're not sure about the health of your sex partner. In the future, close your eyes tightly when he shoots his load in the direction of your chest or face, or if you're up for a little sexy scientist role-playing, wear lab goggles!

TIPS ON MAKING CUM TASTE BETTER

Scientists haven't yet undertaken an experiment to determine whether diet affects the flavor of his semen, although most people believe it does. (This holds true for women's lubrications, too!) We suppose a laboratory-style test of this hypothesis could pose some serious challenges. Ultimately, it's up to you to experiment on your own and decide whether pineapple (or anything else) truly makes his pudding taste sweeter.

If you are the type of girl who likes to swallow but sometimes gets offended by the flavor of his spunk, here are a few fun ways to take the ick out of his love stick.

Shoot It Like Tequila, or an Oyster!

Just because you swallow doesn't mean you have to swish the stuff around in your mouth like you would a mouthful of fine Malbec. When he ejaculates, simply push the head of his cock past your taste buds toward the back of your throat and swallow it down. No muss, no fuss.

Add Your Own Flavor

Try sucking on a lollipop or a mint before (or even during) a blow job, or coat his shaft (avoiding his meatus) with a powdered candy such as Pop Rocks or Fun Dips. But don't use mouthwash, chili peppers, or lemons, as these can irritate his penis, and don't chew gum during a blow job, or you'll run the risk of accidentally chomping down on him! As a safe but not necessarily as tasty alternative, try one of the many varieties of flavored lubrication and powders available at sex toy stores.

Taste Is in the Nose

If you've ever had a stuffy nose, you know the effect that your sense of smell has on your taste buds. Try experimenting with this interaction by placing a drop of perfume on your upper lip, or filling the room with scented candles or the scent of homemade cinnamon rolls. You may find that the pleasing smells filling your nose will make his cum shot that much more palatable. You can also try to not breathe through your nose when you swallow, but we don't advise you to wear an unseemly looking nose plug or pinch your nose with your fingers while you are going down on him.

An Acquired Taste

Once you've been with your partner for some time, you should become accustomed to and perhaps even enjoy the way he tastes. Think of his semen as being like sophisticated hors d'oeuvres at a fancy French restaurant; it's an acquired taste.

THE PRACTICAL SIDE OF SEMEN: CONCEPTION

Indeed, it is fun to squirt his juice on your boobs, or surprise him by swallowing it down like a naughty girl. But the ultimate purpose of semen is to produce itty-bitty babies that turn into cute kids, and then evil teens, and eventually, responsible, well-rounded adults who could someday be president.

Out of the millions of sperm in each glorious ejaculation, it only takes one victorious swimmer to conceive; however, sometimes finding that singular little guy is a challenge (unless of course you are *not* trying to get pregnant, which miraculously makes getting knocked up as easy as ordering pizza). If you are looking to conceive, here are some important tips to help make sure that your guy's magic sauce is in tip-top baby-making shape.

Limit His Time in the Hot Tub

There is a reason that his scrotum keeps such careful tabs on the temperature of his testicles. If his nuts get too hot (98°F/37°C or warmer), they turn into lazy good-for-nothings and put a halt on sperm production. Spending thirty minutes or more in a hot tub can lower his sperm count for months, since it takes about three months for his body to produce these wonder worms. Note that this rule only pertains to direct heat applied to his crotch.

Avoid Drinking Alcohol and Smoking Cigarettes

Research has found that both alcohol and cigarettes negatively impact male fertility. They can cause low sperm count, abnormal/deformed sperm, weak sperm with low motility. If you and your honey are serious about getting pregnant, he should lay off of these vices at least until the magic moment happens.

More Sex, Less Masturbation

We don't want to discourage masturbation, as it is a very healthy practice for him in general. However, if he is dealing with low sperm count when you are trying to conceive, it's helpful if he saves his best batches of baby batter for you. This is especially important around the time you are ovulating. Saving up for sex helps improve the quality of his semen by capitalizing on his sperm reserves.

Technical Difficulties

Some studies indicate that laptops and cell phones may affect his sperm quality. Research has shown that extended cell phone use—four or more hours per day—may decrease sperm count and motility due to the electromagnetic radiation emitted by the devices. However, they admitted that the studies were small and may not be representative of a larger population.

One study found that men who use laptops (and place them on their laps) significantly increase their scrotal temperature. Application of direct heat to the testicles is a proven factor in low sperm count. Researchers concluded that repeated exposure of his lap to his laptop could have a negative impact on fertility, particularly of young men who are more apt to use this technology over a period of many years.

SCIENTIFICALLY SPEAKING—
WHAT IS A VASECTOMY?

For those men who are absolutely positive that they don't want to make any (more) babies, a vasectomy is the most reliable (more than 99 percent effective) and permanent method of male birth control. Although getting a vasectomy is painful, and a lot of men may whine and demand ice cream and full control of the remote during recovery, it's not that big of a deal when compared to other surgical procedures. A vasectomy is performed as an outpatient procedure that takes about a half hour at his doctor's office. The doctor starts by giving a local anesthetic to numb his nuts, then pokes two teeny tiny holes in either side of his scrotum to access the vas deferens tubes (the two ducts that sperm travel down on their way out of his testicles). The doctor cuts a small part of these vas deferens and seals the ends shut; the holes are so small that typically your lover won't need stitches. He'll be sent home with instructions to ice his junk, watch sports, and avoid sex for a couple of weeks.

In a few weeks, your guy will need to jack off into a cup for the laboratory to test for sperm. Before he's cleared for baby-free sex, he'll need to generate two consecutive samples of sperm-free semen, which can take three months or more. After all is said and done, he'll still orgasm and ejaculate as he did before—after all, he's now missing only less than 5 percent of his total ejaculatory fluid. Some men even report heightened arousal, likely because they're no longer afraid of getting you knocked up.

Other Hurdles

It has also been argued that wearing tight underwear, spending a lot of time riding a bicycle, or even sitting for long stretches of time can decrease fertility, as these activities may increase scrotal temperature. It's best for him not to get his tighty whities in a bundle over these habits, unless he's really having serious fertility issues and his doctor suggests he should swap out his briefs for boxers, his bike for jogging shoes, and his desk job for a construction gig.

SEMEN: WHAT IS IT GOOD FOR?

Besides its obvious purpose for procreation, it seems people are always trying to come up with more uses for semen. You might have heard stories that semen is good for your skin, your hair, and your mood. But are they true?

Semen Is an Excellent Hair Product

A hilarious scene from the 1998 movie *There's Something About Mary* depicts Ted (Ben Stiller) jacking off before his date with Mary (Cameron Diaz) and shooting so hard that he gets some ejaculate on his ear. When he opens the door for Mary, she thinks that his jizz is hair gel and, much to the chagrin (or glee) of viewers, proceeds to scoop it off his ear and rub it in her pretty, blond locks.

It turns out she's not the only woman who has put semen in her hair. In 2008, the swank Hari's Hair & Beauty salon in London offered a hair treatment that was said to nourish and revitalize the hair. The secret ingredient? Bull semen. For a while it was the trendiest treatment in London, with women paying over $100 to have their hair coated in bovine spooge. The idea was that the protein punch delivered by the semen would make hair stronger and shinier and even help it grow. However, Hari has since taken chilled bull semen off the menu and replaced it with a less offensive keratin and avocado oil treatment.

Semen Is Good for Your Skin

Proponents of using semen as a moisturizer argue that the solution contains vitamins and salts (from the urethra) that give you a glowing complexion. However, results have been inconclusive.

While it can be fun to allow your partner to ejaculate on your boobs in the heat of excitement, don't worry about massaging it into your skin. It's probably best to wipe it off, or hop in a nice steamy shower and wash it off after playtime.

Semen Is an Antidepressant

Researchers at the State University of New York at Albany found that females who had sex without condoms were less depressed than their safer-sex-practicing counterparts. They discovered that "not only were females who were having sex without condoms less depressed, but depressive symptoms and suicide attempts among females who used condoms were proportional to the consistency of condom use." They also said women who don't use condoms become more depressed the longer they waited between sexual encounters.

Whether this is true or not, we think that contracting an STI or having an unwanted pregnancy would be much more depressing than using condoms. It's also important to note that, even though the condom users scored higher than their condom-free counterparts on the Beck Depression Inventory scale, most of them didn't even score high enough to be considered moderately depressed.

Semen Contains Vitamins

According to sex therapist Dr. Jenni Skyler, a teaspoon of semen contains about five calories and is made up of fructose sugar, water, vitamin C, citric acid, protein, and zinc. She says, "Because the calories are so few, the amount of each ingredient is almost microscopic. So, don't worry about packing on the pounds if you swallow a little semen, and certainly don't depend on it for any kind of nutritional enhancement."

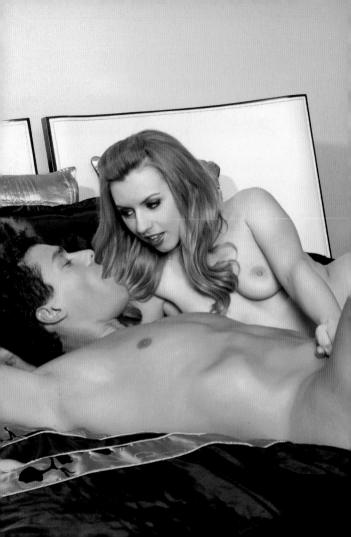

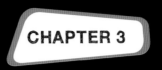

CHAPTER 3

PLAYING WITH DICK: SEXY WAYS TO HANDLE HIS HARD-ON

Now it's time to play with his favorite plaything as if it were yours. Part of becoming a true penis genius is learning and applying exciting, orgasm-inducing techniques. Here are the sexiest ways to handle his hard-on using hand jobs, blow jobs, sex positions, and, yes, even sex toys.

Before we get started, there are a few ground rules:

❶ Always practice safe sex. Unless you are drug- and disease-free and in a monogamous, long-term relationship, use condoms!

❷ After learning all the tips and tricks in the book, remember that every man is different. What has one man spilling spoons full of population pudding onto your bedspread may have another yawning and scratching his nuts. To ensure your sexual success, communicate and find out what your guy wants and needs in the sack.

❸ Remember to ask for his permission, especially when trying new or unusual techniques. If he's never used a cock ring, it would be best to present it to him to inspect before just slipping it over his pecker like a surprise engagement ring. Nothing is worse than being rejected because he's unpleasantly shocked by your explorations.

❹ Keep an open mind and have fun! Sometimes new techniques can induce giggling fits, while others can induce fits of ejaculation. If at first you don't suck-seed, try, try again.

GIVING FANTASTIC FELLATIO

Almost every woman today has given at least a little head in her life. In fact, get a little wine in your best girlfriends, and more than likely you'll have more than a few of them boasting, "I give the best blow jobs in the world!" (And more power to the empowered cocksuckers out there!) But whether you're a novice or a connoisseur, there are always a few new signature moves you can put in your oral arsenal.

The Rules

There are a few ground rules to follow when it comes to mouth-on-cock action. Follow these and you're already halfway there to being a great blow job giver:

❶ **You have to enjoy it.** One of the most frequent comments we hear from men regarding blow jobs is, if he can tell you don't like being on the giving end, it's difficult for him to enjoy being on the receiving end. Says Dave, a thirty-eight-year-old attorney, "For me to get off during a BJ, she has to enjoy it. If you don't enjoy it, don't waste my time and yours." So, unless he has a kink for having you do things you really don't enjoy, approach the blow job as the sexy, playful, and pleasure-giving act it's meant to be. (And for those of you who are reluctant to apply mouth to cock, we offer a few tips later.)

❷ **No biting!** Another thing on which men universally agree: Biting is a big no-no when it comes to his penis. So ladies, save the bite marks for his neck.

Tips to Try If the Blow Job Isn't Your Thing (Yet)

There are a few ground rules to follow when it comes to mouth-on-cock action. Follow these and you're already halfway to being a great blow job giver:

❶ **Start in the shower.** Many women worry about cleanliness. The solution? Take the cleaning routine into your own hands. Washing him gently is also a great way to get him primed for your lip and tongue action. You can even start the sucking right in the shower. Just turn the shower nozzle so you don't get streams of water on your face while you're going down.

❷ Try small licks and soft kisses. If the thought of taking his entire member into your mouth and sucking like a vacuum is intimidating, start out small with a few tender licks on his cockhead and a trail of sweet kisses down the shaft. When you see how much he enjoys your ministrations, you may be inspired to do a little more each time. You can build your blow job technique in stages and at your own pace.

❸ Use the other tools at your disposal. You don't have to gag yourself to make him feel like he's getting some great head. If you're just not feeling up to using your tongue and mouth to get the whole job done, feel free to use your hands or any other body part to help you out. Swirl your tongue around the head of his cock as you stroke his shaft with your well-lubricated fingers or even a vibrating toy. Remember: The shaft responds to pressure, so while you're sucking his head you can use your hands to simulate the sensations of sex.

Tips to Try If You're Proficient in Penis-Sucking

❶ Use your tongue. It's not all about sucking and swallowing. The tongue is what makes the mouth a unique giver of pleasure. After all, no other body part is equipped with this dexterous little muscle. While giving him a blow job, use it to your advantage!

Try pushing his head into your mouth and leaving your lips loose enough so that you can use your tongue to flick his shaft, alternating from the right, left, and lower sides of his cock. Use your tongue like a corkscrew to swirl around his head and upper shaft (watch your teeth when using this technique). You can also use your tongue to stroke his frenulum, the highly sensitive area right under the cockhead on the underside of his penis. Or hold the top side of his penis in one hand and lap the underside in long, sensuous licks from his testicles to the tip of his dick and back again.

❷ Love him with your lips. Lavish your guy with chaste, angelic kisses. Start at his belly button, kiss down his treasure trail, around his cockhead, down his shaft, and along his testicles. Wear bright red lipstick and leave a trail as you go.

❸ Add a touch of vibration. When his cock is sliding into your mouth, make long, low, moaning sounds. If you let them reverberate through your throat, they'll add just a touch of a vibrating sensation, which can be quite tantalizing for him. Not to mention that most men love to hear a woman moan—auditory stimulation like this will make the blow job that much hotter.

❹ Tickle with the teeth. This technique is for the more advanced cocksucker. After all, you have to learn and obey the rules before you can break them. While keeping the "no teeth" rule in mind, be aware that some men enjoy a little bit of toothy stimulation on the shaft—far, far away from the more sensitive head. This is much more of a teeth-tickle than a bite and takes a very light touch.

If your guy is one of these adventurous few, push his cockhead to the back of your mouth and gently graze the skin of his shaft with your teeth. Keep it under control, though; you don't want to accidentally clamp down.

❺ Deep throating. This "holy grail" move in the world of cocksucking takes some practice, mainly because of that pesky gag reflex. True deep throating involves pushing the head of his cock past the uvula (the tear-drop shaped tissue that hangs down at the back of your mouth) and into your throat. While you might not make it this far, even taking his cock in as far as you are able is enough to drive most guys out of their minds.

The key is to relax, get in a position where your neck is extended (lying with your head off the edge of a bed works best), extend your tongue as far as you can, and slowly draw his penis inside as far as you are able. In this position, it will be hard for you to control the sucking motion, and it may involve your guy thrusting into your mouth. Stay calm and let him control the motions.

Lubricant is critical, and sometimes saliva just isn't enough. Porn stars use a product called Albolene, which is actually a makeup remover, but it's nontoxic, tasteless, and super-slippery. You can also try numbing your throat with Chloraseptic spray. Our gag reflexes are least active in the morning, so this may be a fun way to start your day.

❻ It's a team effort. While we might separate blow jobs from hand jobs, a finger in the butt from hands on the nuts, the truth is all of these sex acts can work together as a team. Many of the men we surveyed told us that the surest way to bring them off (outside of intercourse) is by mixing all these techniques into one giant climactic bomb.

❼ 69 is divine. For mutual satisfaction there is, simply put, nothing better than 69. In this position, you are both mouth to genitals, allowing for the simultaneous giving and receiving of oral pleasure. A great advantage of 69 is sometimes you can get so lost in the pleasure you are receiving that you lose your pesky gag reflex.

To get the most from this classic position, experiment with variations. Try him on top, you on top, or both of you lying sideways nose to crotch. For a real twist, have your guy lie down with his feet dangling off the edge of the bed, and climb on top. Then have him sit up, keeping his mouth on your pussy and yours on his cock. You'll now be inverted, so use your hands on the edge of the bed to support your weight. If he's really strong, wrap your hands around his backside and have him stand up while in position. The head rush you'll get from being upside down will make your orgasm that much more delightful.

GET A HANDLE ON HAND JOBS

Want to wrap him around your finger? Giving a hand job is a simple and fun way to excite your man, make him extra hard, and bring him to a hands-on climax. Just as with the blow job, some girls love giving a hand job and some girls could care less. To all those with friendly fingers out there, we'd like to point out that hand jobs are the go-to move when you want to be discreet (think sexy situations in which you can't remove your own clothing or properly bend over for a nice, sloppy BJ), and they're also perfect for when you want to practice safe sex but don't have a condom.

The Rules

If you can understand and follow these ground rules for jerking him off, he's that much closer to being putty in your hands:

❶ **Take care of your mitts**. Make sure your hands are not overly dry, cracked, or calloused. We don't want to chafe the poor guy!

❷ **The pleasures of lube**. When giving hand jobs, try your favorite sex lube, suntan lotion, or sudsy soap in the shower. While lube isn't always necessary, it can be lots of fun.

❸ **Let him show you how it's done.** Let's face it: Your guy is an expert at stroking his own shaft. What better way to learn how to handle his hard-on than by asking him to masturbate for you? It's even better than having him try to tell you what he likes. Follow his lead and match your man stroke for stroke to bring him to a blissful finish.

Tips to Try If You've Mastered the Basic Stroke

For you ladies who've already mastered masturbating your man, here are some genius tips to add to your repertoire:

❶ **Finger his frenulum and caress his cockhead**. Much like your clit and labia are for you, the frenulum and cockhead (glans) are the most sensitive to touch for him. The frenulum is located on the underside of his shaft; it's that little strip of flesh that connects the top of his shaft to his head. Try gripping his shaft firmly in one hand and pumping up and down, and use your other hand to rub his glans in circles. Gently tease the area with your fingernails, or use your thumb to stroke his frenulum in a short, rhythmic, upward motion from the bottom of the strip to the top.

❷ **Use different strokes**. Don't feel like you have to stick to the predictable, basic up-and-down stroke. A little creativity in your touch can be a nice surprise that can bring him to the brink.

❸ **Try adding a _twist_**: Instead of stroking in straight lines, wrap your slippery palm around his shaft and twist your wrist left and right as you simultaneously stroke up and down.

Or try forming a tight _ring_ with your thumb and forefinger and push his cockhead through your lubed-up digits. Focus on squeezing his coronal ridge through the tightened space you've made with your fingers while using your other hand to caress his balls.

Tease his shaft with light brushes of your fingertips: Place your palm on his cockhead and let your fingers graze up and down his shaft, just lightly scratching the surface.

Using a firm grip, wrap your hand around his shaft, beneath the glans, and squeeze and release him in a rhythmic pulse. Do not stroke your hand up and down. Use your tongue or your other hand to caress his exposed cockhead or massage his testicles while you push him to the edge.

❹ **Try some shower fun**. Bring a little thrill to your morning shower by popping in with him while he is warm, wet, and sudsy. For a slippery encounter, use body soap (avoid shampoo) or a few drops of silicone lube. Stand behind him, reach around to take his

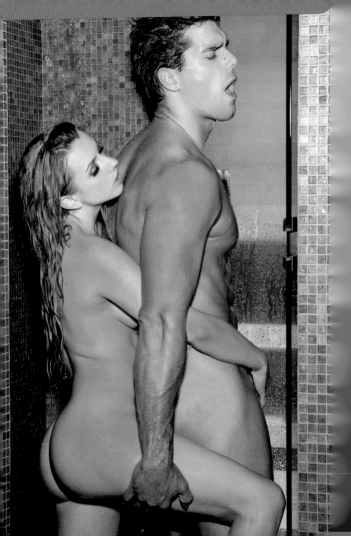

penis in your hands, and give him a nice rhythmic massage while rubbing your breasts against his back. Keep at it until he spouts, and it will be the perfect start to his workday.

Tips to Try If the Hand Job Just Doesn't Sound Hot

If you think hand jobs sound boring or are too much work, have we got news for you! There are many ways to make slipping his penis between your palms exciting and fun:

❶ Be spontaneous. Giving a hand job is the perfect sex act for spontaneous fun, as it doesn't require much undressing and can be done quite surreptitiously. If you find yourself in a situation where you don't have any lube (say, in the back row of a nearly empty movie theater), it is still possible to give a knockout hand job. Simply use a featherlight touch. The skin on his penis is much more elastic than you might think, and you can move it without hurting him. Be aware, if you go the lube-free route; make sure you're not stroking him with chapped fingers after a day of rock climbing or gardening without gloves. While lube isn't necessary, your soft skin on his is a must.

❷ Remember, you don't have to use your hand from beginning to end. Once you've had fun wrapping your fingers around him, you can always switch to a blow job or intercourse to make him come.

SEXCITING POSITIONS TO BRING TO THE BEDROOM

When it comes to sex positions, the majority of men we surveyed prefer Doggy-Style (you on your hands and knees with him penetrating from behind) above all others, followed by Cowgirl (you on top) and Missionary (him on top). Sure, these may be great go-to positions to ensure a satisfying orgasm. But what would happen if you tried something new? We challenge you to try these five fabulous positions that will stimulate his penis in different ways. (For additional positions tailored to the size and shape of your man's package, read chapter six.)

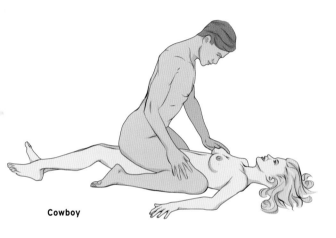

Cowboy

Position #1: Cowboy

If he loves Cowgirl and Missionary, he might just love Cowboy! This position combines the two for penis-pleasing fun. Lie on your back and spread your legs. He straddles your hips on his knees, while keeping his body upright, and penetrates you. Once he's comfortably inside, close your legs for a nice, tight squeeze. This will give you the feeling of fullness, and he'll have the luxury of being able to control the thrusts and spur his way to a powerful climax.

Position #2: Cuban Plunge

Here's a spicy twist on Missionary: the Cuban Plunge. Start in
Missionary and then bring your knees up to your chest, letting
your calves rest on his shoulders. This position allows extra-deep
penetration, so don't be surprised if you feel his little head bump up
against your back wall. For a little added fun, reach around your
thighs and give his testicles a massage as he plunges away.

Position #3: Superwoman

Take Doggy-Style up a notch and try Superwoman. Stand and face
the edge of the bed (or another sturdy, flat surface, such as your
dining room table) and bend over it. Support your torso on the

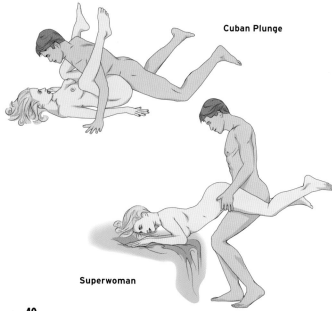

Cuban Plunge

Superwoman

40

surface and extend your legs in the air behind you so you are positioned like a flying superhero. Your partner enters from between your legs and supports your hips with his arms. Because Superwoman requires a bit of core strength and leg stamina on your part, it can be made easier by doing it in a place where you can push your feet up against a wall. This position is great for his thrusting control, and gives you the delightful feeling of being completely ravished by your man.

Position #4: Amazon

Let your wild side out to explore the Amazon position. This girl-on-top arrangement will give your man a whole world of new sensations. He lies on his back and draws his knees up to his chest, with his legs slightly spread. You can either squat (if you're strong) or kneel (if your legs tire easily) on either side of his hips and slide onto his cock. Place pillows under your knees if you are too short for this position. The Amazon may make him feel vulnerable, as it completely exposes his nether regions to you, plus he'll have to let you take control because he'll have to let you take control because he'll be pinned beneath you. He can caress your tits or tease your clit as you ride him. You can easily reach around to caress his perineum or anus, as well. Also, this is a great position for G-spot stimulation, and because you'll be controlling the thrust and depth of penetration, it's a good go-to move for when you are ready to achieve your orgasm.

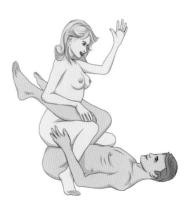

Amazon

Bookends

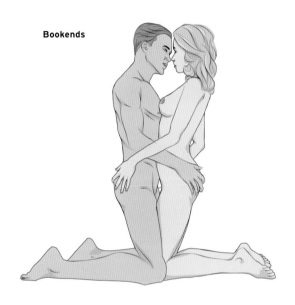

Position #5: Bookends

After reading a bit of erotica together, you may want to continue your own sex story by trying Bookends. Kneel facing each other. Spread your legs and have him thrust up into you. If he is much taller than you, he may have to spread his legs wider than yours so he can enter you from below. You can either keep your knees wide for a smooth entry, or squeeze them together to add some friction. Take advantage of being face-to-face by kissing each other and massaging each other's nipples, shoulders, and backs.

THE JOYS OF SEX TOYS

Masturbation sleeves and cock rings are two categories of sex toys that are made specifically for the penis and can be lots o' fun during playtime. Remember, while he can use these toys during his solo explorations, they're also a great way to add a kinky twist to your partnered sex.

Masturbation Sleeves

Just like your dildo is meant to simulate a penis, masturbation sleeves are designed to simulate a vagina or anus. He uses one by lubing up his penis, slipping the sleeve on, and pumping it up and down his shaft. The devices come in an array of materials, from silicone to ultra-realistic skinlike material. Your guy can choose from sleeve models that range from toylike, colorful tubes to realistic body parts modeled after porn stars. Sleeves are also equipped with different textured interiors, including smooth, ribbed, and wavy, which lend variety to the sensations.

However, be aware that one size does not necessarily fit all, especially if your man is on the larger side of the spectrum. Sophisticated sex toy sites have sizing charts to help you determine which sleeve will best fit your man's equipment. With all the variety out there, it may take you a few tries before you find his perfect match.

Some masturbation sleeves come with their own set of humorous issues, too. Karl, a thirty-four-year-old electrical engineer, says of his toy, "My girlfriend bought me a masturbation sleeve, and it almost feels like the real thing and it's a nice change-up from using my hand. But I don't use it much because my jizz squirts out the opening when I ejaculate, and then I have to go find where it landed." An easy way to solve this messy problem is to have him wear a condom, or you can squeeze the end of the tube closed or put your palm over the top of his head when he comes. Or look for a model that has a closed-off end.

Cock Rings

A cock ring is a delightful device to bring into the bedroom. Traditional cock rings are made of metal or rubber, but newer models come in a multitude of materials with a variety of features and textures. They work by trapping the blood in his penis, which results in larger and longer-lasting erections, so they are particularly handy for guys who worry about the size of their peckers or premature ejaculation.

The key is choosing the right size. The smaller diameter rings trap more blood in his penis, causing more intense erections. But a cock ring novice may freak out when asked to slip his dick into something that looks a lot smaller than his shaft. When you buy his first cock ring, choose a ring that is about the same diameter as his erection (a 1.75- to 2-inch [4.4- to 5-centimeter] ring will fit most men). Once he becomes more experienced, he can try something smaller. Don't leave a cock ring on for longer than about twenty minutes at a time, as extended wear can cause nerve damage. Be sure to remove it if he feels any pain or his penis or testicles become cold.

A cock ring should be put on when your man is still flaccid. He should apply a generous amount of lube to his shaft and balls, and then slide the ring all the way to the base of his cock and gently pull his testicles through. If he is wary of pulling his testicles through the ring, he can simply wear it at the base of the shaft (although once things get slippery, it may slide off during intercourse). If he's working himself into a metal ring, have him put his testicles in first, one at a time, and then push his flaccid penis through. Another option is to buy a ring that has an opening snap; this way he can just button up after it's on. Be aware that if he gets too excited, there is a chance that the snap will pop open and the ring could fall off during play.

For extra sensation, try using a vibrating cock ring. Just position the vibrating attachment so that it contacts your clit.

Sometimes all it takes to add more excitement to your penis handling is adding a little variety to your routine. Trying new positions and techniques, and adding new props to your repertoire, will take you from being a penis layperson to a penis expert.

SCIENTIFICALLY SPEAKING—
WHICH LUBE SHOULD I USE?

Here's a handy chart to use when picking out the appropriate lube.

	Water-based, no glycerin	Flavored or warming water-based	Silicone-based	Petroleum oil-based
Pros/Cons	Very safe and have multiple uses, but dry out quickly and need to be reapplied frequently	Adds fun sensations, but many flavored/warming lubes contain glycerin, which can cause yeast infections	Is great for water play, is long lasting, but damages certain materials and can stain your sheets	Never dries out, is long lasting, but damages certain materials and can stain your sheets
Vaginal Sex	YES	NO	YES	NO
Oral Sex	YES	YES	NO	NO
Anal Sex	YES	YES	YES	NO
Hand Jobs/ Male Masturbation	YES	YES	YES	YES
Latex Condoms	YES	YES	YES	NO
Silicon Toys	YES	YES	NO	NO
Rubber, Metal, Glass, or Wood Toys	YES	YES	YES	YES

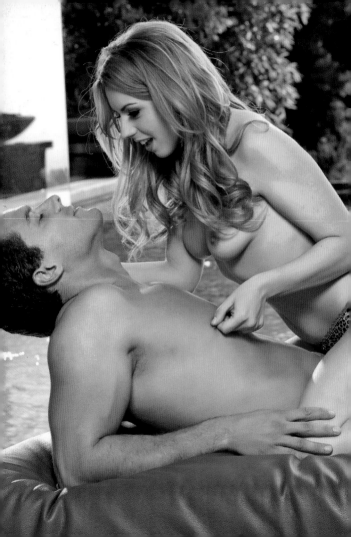

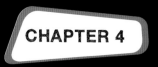

CHAPTER 4

PENIS TEASE: PUSHING HIS OTHER BUTTONS

Ladies, we all know that men are more than just the sum of their penis parts, right? So, it makes sense that being a true penis genius means also understanding some of his other buttons, and knowing when and how to push them. These buttons include the nipples, the perineum, the testicles, the prostate, and the anus, and they are all connected to his sexual arousal. Let's talk about how and when to touch these private places in conjunction with your penis play.

TANTALIZE HIS TESTICLES

Testicles reside in the scrotal sack that hangs just below his penis. At first glance, they may look as foreign as those furry monsters from *Fraggle Rock*, but as a major center of male pleasure, it would do you well to become acquainted with these little guys.

In our survey, a whopping 56 percent of men reported that they love having their testicles stimulated, especially in conjunction with intercourse.

Sexy Techniques to Try

❶ Incorporate the testicles into your blow job technique. Give them a tender squeeze or lube up and massage them very gently in your palm as you tongue his shaft.

❷ Try gently tugging down on the testicles in a milking motion. Some men love the feeling of having the scrotum and balls gently stretched. Be sure to ask him if he likes it.

❸ Use a feather or your fingernails to tickle and tease.

❹ Lap each testicle with your tongue, one at a time, and then oh-so-gently bring one into your mouth with your lips and tongue. Suckle it in your mouth before you release it, and do the same to the other one.

(For more ideas, see chapter one.)

Contraindication Warning

The testicles are extremely sensitive to pain (just as your ovaries would be if they had to hang outside the body). Never poke, knock, or squish them (or it will be a cold shoulder and lights out tonight).

RIDE THE PERINEUM HIGHWAY

The perineum is that little stretch of pleasurable highway that runs from his anus to just behind his ball sack. The subcutaneous tissue is sensitive, smooth, and rife with nerve endings. Because it's located below his cock and balls, it's one spot that is easily overlooked. However, men love to have this erogenous zone licked, fingered, and massaged. Forty-four percent of the men we surveyed say they enjoy having their perineum stimulated during sex.

Sexy Techniques to Try

❶ To spice up that hand job, gently cup and lift his testicles with one hand as you stroke his shaft with the other. Flatten your tongue and gently lap the length of his perineum, from the edge of his anus to the base of his scrotum. Repeat.

❷ Next time you are riding on top like a naughty cowgirl, reach between his legs and place one or two fingers on this lovely morsel of flesh and stroke in circular motions. When you can tell he's close to the brink, use your knuckle to increase the pressure and massage the spot like you're kneading a sexy piece of guy-dough. Be careful not to press too hard, though—you don't want to hurt him.

❸ For a completely out-of-this-world sensation, invest in a small vibrating bullet and roll it against his perineum while giving him head. Start at a low-level vibration and if he responds with pleasure, turn it up until you slingshot him to the moon.

THE BACKDOOR MAN

In our survey, 42 percent of men reported that they enjoy a woman who plays with their butthole. Because this secret space has a large number of nerve endings, the anus is a hugely sensitive erogenous area. Now don't be shy ladies. If your lover loves a little backdoor action, or is even curious about it, just a brush of your finger against the opening can be enough to send some men into la-la land.

Sexy Techniques to Try

❶ As you deliver that knockout blow job, gently press the pad of your finger against his anal opening. You can just let your digit rest there, or slowly massage his pucker-hole in circles. Try timing these with the circular swirls of your tongue.

❷ If you are a bit more adventurous, take a good dollop of silicone or water-based lube and gently explore around the opening before pushing your finger inside. (Be sure you have clipped your nails short and smooth!) Press against the walls of his anus and slowly open the area to your touch. Press your finger in a couple of inches. If you are overcome with the desire to finger-fuck him, make sure you ask him first and go slowly.

❸ To kick it up a notch, once he's relaxed to your fingers, slip in a sex toy specifically designed for his butt. Anal beads, butt plugs, and slim dildos designed just for anal penetration are among the toys you might want to stock in your bedside drawer. Be sure that whatever you choose has a wide base or a handle. There is no back wall to the anal canal, and a toy that is not designed for anal pleasure could potentially get lost up there.

MASSAGE HIS PROSTATE

The prostate can be a source of intense and unique erotic pleasure. When a man ejaculates, the prostate contracts, pulses, and expels the fluid that makes up about a third of his semen. When you massage his prostate (with his permission) by way of his perineum or rectum, you not only stimulate the many nerve endings that surround his prostate, but also encourage and enhance the pleasurable orgasmic contraction. The intensity of his orgasm can be increased two- to threefold with prostate massage.

Follow These Simple Steps for a Perfect Prostate Massage

❶ Clip your fingernails; nothing is worse than a sharp object up the butt.

❷ Have him clean thoroughly.

❸ Slick him up with water- or silicone-based lube.

❹ Loosen him up and get him excited by kissing him, playing with his penis, and massaging his perineum and anal opening.

❺ Once he's relaxed, slowly push your finger into his tush up to your first knuckle. The pad of your finger should be facing the front side of his body.

❻ Feel around for hard tissue, about the size of a walnut. That's his prostate. When you find it, begin to stroke it by making a "come hither" type of gesture.

❼ Continue to play with his cock, kiss him, and encourage him to enjoy himself. You'll know that you've hit jackpot when he starts to pulse around your finger—the beginning contractions of his ejaculation.

TITILLATE HIS NIPPLES

In our survey, 61 percent of men reported that their nipples are a particularly sensitive erogenous zone, and 23 percent enjoy nipple stimulation during sex. Touch his nipples in the same way you enjoy having yours touched.

Sexy Techniques to Try

❶ Pinch the nub gently between your thumb and forefinger, and then rotate your fingers clockwise and counterclockwise; ask him if he wants more or less pressure.

❷ Roll the nipple under the palm of your hand.

❸ Pinch his nipples lightly (or firmly) between your fingers and tug on them, or even bite them.

❹ Lick and suck those babies to erection.

❺ Rest your hands on his chest and, using just your thumbs, rub his nipples in an upward stroke from bottom to top.

❻ If you are both feeling particularly adventurous, try using one of the various nipple-teasing toys available at sex toy stores. Many of them come with suctioning, vibrating, or pinching action. Just secure one of these little suckers onto his nips, and your hands and mouth will be free to go to town on the rest of his body.

Which parts of the body do you like to have stimulated during intercourse?

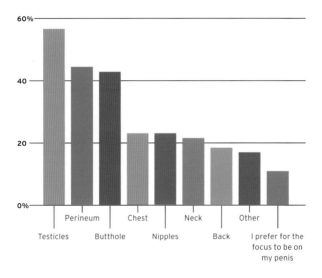

Fifty-six percent of our men say they love having their testicles played with during intercourse. What's in the "Other" category? Abs, prostate, legs, ears, and feet.

EROTIC MASSAGE: A ROLE-PLAYING GAME

An erotic massage can be just what the doctor ordered. Add a little role-playing to this activity to make it a truly sexy experience.

Here is how the story might go: Pretend you are a professional massage therapist, and your lover is a new customer. Set up a massage area on your bed; be sure to cover it with a towel or a set of sheets that you don't mind spilling a little oil on. Set up the room with dim lights and inviting music. Instruct your "customer" to fully undress and lie face down beneath the sheet, and then leave the room. When he is situated, politely knock on the door and return to the room.

Start by folding the sheet down to expose his back, leaving his buttocks covered. Gently stroke his back with your fingertips. Ask him where he is holding tension. Get to know him a little–ask him what he does for a living and whether he is in a relationship. Tell him he has a sexy back. Ask him if he lifts weights. Pour a tablespoon of massage oil onto your hands and rub them together to warm it up. Slather it onto his skin. Ask him how it feels. Start to massage it in, rubbing up and down his spine and in circles around his back and shoulders. Ask him if it's okay to rub his butt, and then slowly pull the sheet down to expose it. Add more oil and begin to rub his behind, kneading it with your knuckles and squeezing it in your fingers. Part his legs and occasionally, "accidentally" brush your fingers against his scrotum and crack. Ask him if he would like to turn over so that you can take care of his front side. When he turns over, massage his chest and abs, but don't touch his penis. Not until he asks you to!

It's a great pleasure to discover all those little off-the-penis parts that give your man a thrill in the sack. Enjoy, be safe, and have fun!

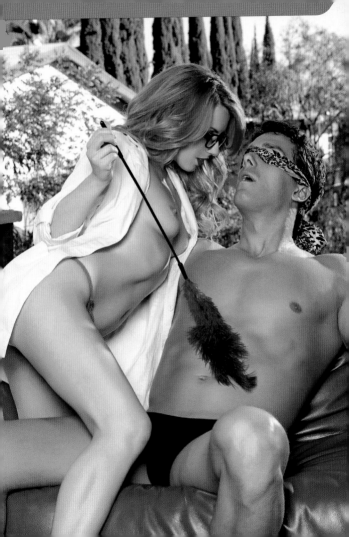

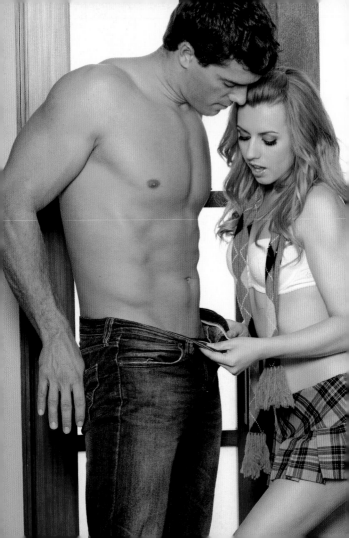

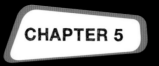

CHAPTER 5

CIRCUMCISED VS. UNCIRCUMCISED: WHAT MODEL DOES YOUR MAN HAVE?

Your man's penis will look, and sometimes react, differently to stimuli based on whether he is circumcised. Do you know what model penis your man has? You might want to take a second look.

Kerri, a thirty-three-year-old electrician, tells us, "My boyfriend and I have been intimate for about three months. It wasn't until recently when I saw his flaccid penis for the first time that I realized that I was dating an uncircumcised man. I've been 'down there' so many times during sex and never noticed his foreskin! It shocked me, but I was pleasantly surprised because I'd heard so many rumors that sex with uncircumcised men was gross. He's actually the best I've ever had. Whether or not it has to do with his intact penis, I'm not sure."

Let's look closely and observe the difference between an uncircumcised cock (**MODEL A**) and a circumcised cock (**MODEL B**).

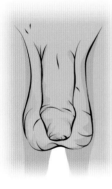

MODEL A

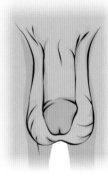

MODEL B

In model A, you'll see when flaccid, the foreskin of the uncircumcised penis completely covers the glans. The urethra of the penis may peek out the end and wink at you, or the foreskin may extend beyond the urethra and look like a deflated balloon.

As his penis hardens under the effects of your genius, you'll notice that the foreskin pulls back and settles under his head, resembling a tube sock. When fully erect, the inner foreskin remains beneath the glans, and the outer layer of the foreskin stretches to the middle of his shaft. Visually, a fully erect, uncut penis looks similar to a cut penis, because the glans is fully visible and the foreskin is taut around the shaft.

In model B, you'll see that a flaccid circumcised penis looks more like a mushroom, with its exposed, helmetlike head. When fully erect, the entire penis fills with blood and expands, making the glans look fuller and the shaft look taut.

WHICH PENIS FEELS MORE PLEASURE?

The argument about which penis feels more pleasure (cut or uncut) continues to be waged in both science and popular culture. Circumcised men argue that having a more exposed glans allows it to be more easily stimulated. Uncircumcised men say that because their glans is protected from daily chafing, when it does come out to play, it's extra sensitive to touch. However, men who've opted to be circumcised later in life have reported a decrease in sensitivity, and these men may be the ones who can give us the best insight into the matter.

With research on the topic mostly inconclusive, it's really anybody's guess as to who feels more pleasure. What we do know from experience is that most men love sex, no matter what model penis they're working with.

WHAT DOES CIRCUMCISION MEAN FOR YOUR SEX LIFE?

What are the differences between playing with a cut versus an uncut cock? While some women can hardly distinguish between the two, others are attuned to the different pleasures each has to offer. Here are some of the discrepancies you might notice (that is, if you're paying close attention!).

Circumcision and Hand Jobs

In our survey, 62.3 percent of women reported a noticeable difference when giving hand jobs to uncircumcised verses circumcised cocks. With an intact foreskin, there is little need for lubrication when giving a hand job thanks to the natural lubrication generated by the mucous membranes in the foreskin.

With a circumcised penis, you'll want to lube up your palm so that the shaft slides against the skin of your hand, or you can use a featherlight touch. With an uncircumcised penis, the foreskin generates its own lube and glides easily along the shaft as if it were a natural masturbation sleeve; all you have to do is slide it up and down. (For more information on giving great hand jobs, see chapter three.)

Circumcision and Giving Head

The biggest complaint women report when it comes to giving head is that sometimes a man doesn't keep his junk nice and clean. Cleanliness is sexiness. This is true whether a man is circumcised or not; after all, your tongue and nose are so involved in the oral experience, a tasty and yummy smelling gent is always preferable.

Uncircumcised men naturally generate a pungent substance called smegma (women produce the same secretion around their labia and clit). Smegma is made from shed skin cells and body secretions and acts as a natural lubricant. When it first develops, it's often clear or whitish and moist and smooth, but if it's allowed to build up, it becomes more of a chunky, cheesy substance. If your lover is uncut, he should bathe and wash regularly and know how to pull the foreskin back to clean out the area.

Let's assume you dive into his drawers and he's sporting a squeaky-clean woody. More than half (53.7 percent) of women we surveyed say they can tell a big difference when giving head to an uncircumcised man. You can bring unique sensations to your uncut man. The opening of the foreskin is particularly sensitive, and a good tease with your tongue into the entrance can cause bedroom earthquakes. Some men like it when you pull the foreskin all the way down before giving oral (this gives you full access to his glans and frenulum), while other men find their glans to be supersensitive, so they prefer you to suck on the foreskin or just be extra-gentle with the head.

Other women are smitten with the circumcised option. Says Lori, a thirtysomething upholsterer, "When giving head, I have found that the head of the circumcised penis is slightly less sensitive than an uncircumcised penis. I personally prefer circumcised penises because they offer a more tactile experience when giving head, as there is never any excess skin." The sensitive frenulum and coronal ridge are fully exposed on circumcised men, and they just beg for you to lick and love them as part of your oral play. (For more information on giving great head, read chapter three.)

Circumcision and Intercourse
In our survey, 65 percent of women say they feel no difference between cut and uncut cock during intercourse. Perhaps this is because our vaginas aren't as discriminating as our fingertips and tongues. However, 18.5 percent say there is something to it. Word on the street indicates that the uncircumcised man's penis is a bit more sensitive than his circumcised counterpart, especially around his glans. Women report that the extra sensitivity leads uncircumcised men to use slower, gentler strokes.

However, other women prefer the action they receive from their uncircumcised lovers. Says Trish, a forty-three-year-old accounting executive, "Being English, I've been with uncircumcised men for most of my life. When I met my current (American) partner, I was delighted with the absolute rough sex he gives me. He seems to need more friction, and uses rapid strokes that drive me absolutely bananas."

Just like size, shape, angle, and function, the foreskin or lack thereof is yet another characteristic that makes your man's cock unique. Whatever you find behind your man's zipper, you should learn about, experiment with, and enjoy his unique pleasure potential.

WHERE DID CIRCUMCISION ORIGINATE?

Circumcision has been in practice for thousands of years. Egyptians left evidence as early as 2300 BC that they performed male genital alteration rituals as a rite of passage at the onset of puberty. Jews continue the practice of circumcision as a religious covenant that harks back to biblical days. Muslim tradition also honors circumcision, as the prophet Mohammed (who, according to some legends, was born without a foreskin) taught that circumcision is customary for men. A popular reason that many nonreligious fathers opt to circumcise their sons is so that their babies will look as they do. Circumcision has maintained its popularity in the United States, while most other Western countries have all but abandoned the practice.

In the United States, circumcision has been routinely performed in hospitals since about 1930. Circumcision peaked in 1975 when about 93 percent of newborn boys were cut; today that number is down to about 80 percent. In Europe, only about 1 percent of newborns are circumcised. Today, circumcision is becoming less popular as questions about its benefits have emerged. American Academy of Pediatrics guidelines now say that circumcision is unnecessary, and some health insurers are calling it a "cosmetic procedure," which means they may not cover the cost.

Circumcision is generally considered to be a safe procedure, with reports of less than 1 percent of cases being "botched" jobs. However, as with any body modification surgery, complications can arise, such as hemorrhaging, infections, and scarring.

Ultimately, parents still have the choice when they have a son as to whether to circumcise him. It's important to do your research and make the best decision for you and your family based on medical information as well as your specific religious or cultural considerations.

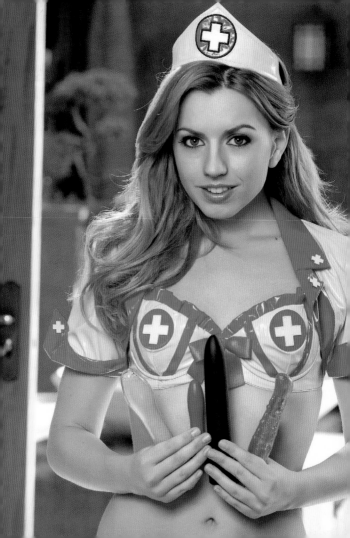

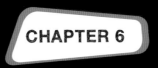

CHAPTER 6

ON SHAPES AND SIZES: PERFECT POSITIONS FOR ALL PENIS PROPORTIONS

Just like fingerprints, no two penises are exactly alike, but most fit into certain broad categories of physical attributes. You may find yourself with a long, slender drink of water, or you may snag yourself a short but rotund specimen. We'll tell you about the best sexual positions you can try to maximize or minimize penetration for the different sizes and shapes of dicks you may come across.

From our conversations with women, we know that each one has her own definition of penis perfection. Some love nothing more than a giant cock, others like a more moderate member, or one with a definite left-hand bend, and still others love whatever comes attached to their sweetheart. It's all a question of how well the two puzzle pieces (yours and his) fit together to maximize mutual pleasure. Says forty-six-year-old K.B., "The best penis for me—in any position—is always the one that's about an inch shorter than my pussy and several inches wider. When we get it all slick and I'm all wet, it feels good to still have to force it a bit to get it in. I have to admit that I hate too-long penises for ANY position. My uterus is happy in her present location. No sense in making the old girl relocate!"

Note that the following penis sizes and suggested positions are generalized examples to try with your partner. It is only through your own exploration that you and your partner(s) will find what works best for your unique anatomies.

THE HULK

(At least 8 inches [20.3 centimeters] in length and 5 inches [12.7 centimeters] in circumference)

Unzipping a man's trousers to discover the Hulk lurking in his boxers (minus the green skin and bad attitude) can be an exciting or an alarming experience, depending on who you are. For some women, there's just nothing as delightful as being filled to capacity (and then some), while other women may find the Hulk intimidating, overwhelming, or just downright painful.

Perfect Positions

If you find that your guy is too large for your dainty parts, try riding him in any variation of the girl-on-top positions, which will allow you to control the depth of his penetration. **Cowgirl** is the most basic of these positions: Your man lies down on a flat surface and you straddle his penis, facing him and keeping your knees on either side of his hips. For a variation, ride him **Reverse Cowgirl**. This position is similar to Cowgirl, but you mount him facing backward so that you are looking at his feet. In this position, he gets a titillating view of your behind. If you require even less of his penis inside while riding, try the **Pearly Gates (page 68-69):** Start in Reverse Cowgirl and then lie back so you are resting against his chest. This will help limit his penetrative range.

Another great option for coupling with a guy who is extremely well-endowed is **Teaspoons.** In this position, you stand on your knees with your legs spread wide. Your guy kneels behind you and penetrates you from behind. This position not only limits his depth and allows you to spread wide enough to accept his girth, but it also gives him the control over thrusting that he won't get with the girl-on-top positions. For a super sexy twist, he can reach around you to rub your clit and play with your breasts.

However, be careful here not to bend over into Doggy Style, which is where you lean forward and put your hands on the floor, as that position provides for incredibly deep penetration and he will be more likely to hit your cervix and the back of your uterus. Ouch!

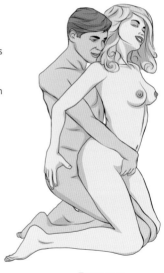

Teaspoons

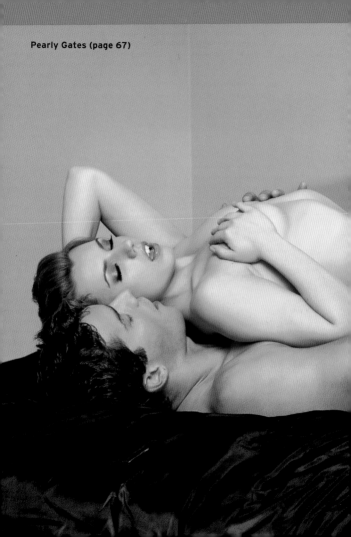

Pearly Gates (page 67)

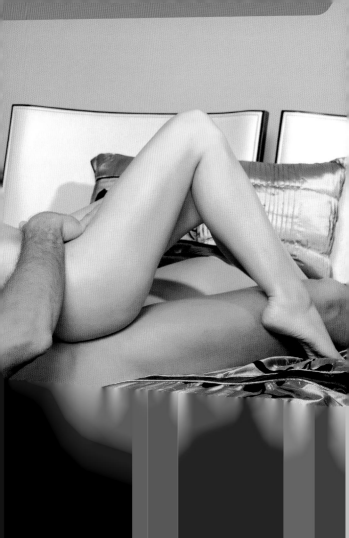

Tasty Tips

For your pleasure, you should be excited and lubricated no matter what size your guy is, but when partnering with the Hulk, it's even more important to be fully aroused. Enjoying a warm-up orgasm via toy play or oral sex prior to penetration can help "loosen" you up and prepare you to accommodate his full size. Amanda, thirty-two, says, "I'm petite and can barely take an average-sized cock. I was recently with a well-endowed man. As long as my mind was on it, he would not fit. He went down on me until I came, held me still enough while I thrashed around, out of my mind, and slipped into me. Well, slipped isn't the right word . . . but before I knew it, there he was."

You can also try slowly stretching yourself during foreplay by using a sequence of toys that range from your ideal size to something close to his size before attempting to accommodate the Hulk. Or ask him to use his fingers to massage and stretch you open beforehand, starting with one digit and graduating up to four fingers. What fun!

And ladies, especially with the Hulk, lubrication is critical. Even if you are dripping wet, we suggest you supplement your natural juices with a healthy dollop of water-based lubrication.

THE TALL DRINK OF WATER

(At least 7 inches [17.8 centimeters] in length and 4 inches [10 centimeters] or thinner in circumference)

These long and slender guys can be a lot of fun to play with, as they are easy to wrap your hand or mouth around, and some women simply love the feel of a long cock inside of them. Just like Rhett Butler, played by the oh-so-drinkable Clark Gable in Gone with the Wind, these guys slide in nice and smooth. But as Scarlett O'Hara knows too well, if you don't handle them properly, they can leave you feeling pricked and stung. That's right, girls, due to the length of the Tall Drink of Water, intercourse brings the risk of painful cervix bumping.

The Jockey

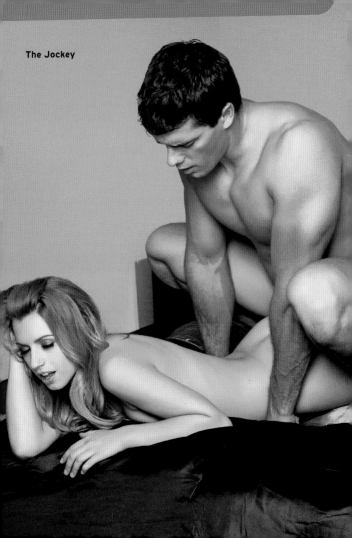

Perfect Positions

Try the **Jockey (page 71):** Start by lying either on your back or your stomach, with your legs spread open. Your guy straddles the outside of your legs and hips in a crouching position, much like that of a jockey (or a certain southern scoundrel we know and love—yum!) riding a racehorse. Let him gently enter you, and then, before he gets too excited and starts thrusting away, squeeze your legs closed around him. This position limits the depth of penetration so you can avoid any uncomfortable bumping sensations, and it also lets him feel fully enveloped because your thighs will press pleasingly around any parts of the shaft that don't make it inside your body. And if his penis is of the super slender variety, having your legs (and pussy) clamped tightly around his cock will provide the luscious sensation that he has additional girth.

Alternatively, ask him to be your **Bodyguard.** With both of you standing, have your guy enter you from behind. If there is a major height difference (you or he) may need to stand on a step or stool (or you can put on your 6-inch stilettos) to attain the right fit. Because he's entering from behind without you being bent over, he can use his length to both of your advantage. Also, this frees up his hands to give you a breast or clit massage. You can reach behind and caress his buttocks as he thrusts his way to bliss.

If his length isn't all that bothersome to you and you've been practicing yoga, ask him to do the **Pile Driver (page 74).** This is one super kinky position that guys of shorter endowments may have trouble accomplishing. In this position, lie on your upper back and raise your lower back and butt off the floor, completely exposing your pussy and pushing your booty skyward. Support your hips with your hands, elbows pressed into the floor. Your knees will fall to either side of your ears. Standing, he straddles you, bending his penis down toward the floor as he enters you. The thrusting motion comes from him squatting and standing as he penetrates. Now he can get to drilling!

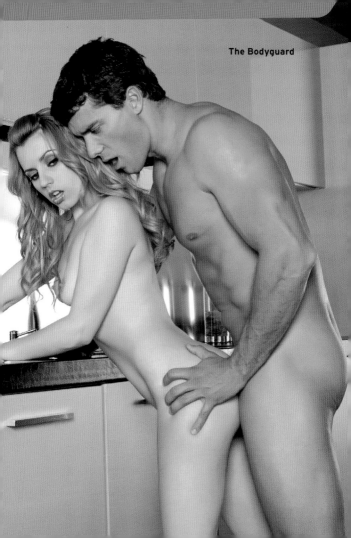

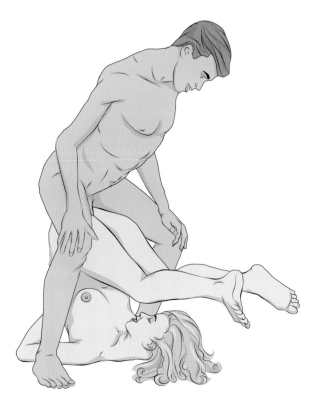

Pile Driver

Tasty Tips

If in any position you try, you find that your guy is so long that he uncomfortably pokes your cervix while thrusting, you can further control the depth of his insertion by wrapping your hand around the base of his penis and giving him a tight squeeze as you ride.

Practicing your Kegels (which you should do no matter what size your guy is) will help you to make the most of the Tall Drink of Water. Tone your vaginal muscles by repetitively squeezing and releasing them. One Kegel consists of both tightening and relaxing the muscle, so begin by tightening your pelvic muscle for three seconds, and relaxing for three seconds. Do ten reps, three times a day. As you get stronger, you can increase the contraction/relaxation time incrementally from three seconds up to ten seconds. The great thing about Kegels is, you can do your reps while sitting at your computer or driving, and nobody will be the wiser! During sex, this strength will help you get a grip around his penis. Doing Kegels also enhances your orgasms, as these are some of the same muscles that contract during your climax.

THE BUBBA

(6.5 inches [16.5 centimeters] or fewer in length and at least 5 inches [12.7 centimeters] in circumference)

The Bubba may be considered the perfect package for those women who love the sensation of being stretched open, yet prefer to have their cervixes left untouched. For yet others, the stretching part may still be a bit of a challenge to overcome.

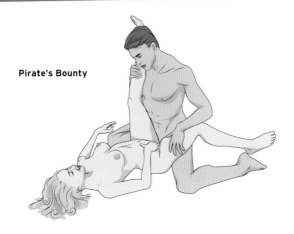

Pirate's Bounty

Perfect Positions

Since controlling depth isn't the issue here, it's best to really open your legs wide for Bubba. The **Missionary** position, and many open-legged variations of Missionary, such as the **Pirate's Bounty** (one leg stretched wide to the side, while the other rests on his shoulder), should provide for perfectly pleasurable penetration. Also, **Standing Doggy** Style, leaning forward over the bed (or your office desk) with your legs spread wide, is a good choice for playing with Bubba.

Tasty Tips

If your vagina is resistant to stretching wide, perform many of the same warm-up exercises described for preparing for the Hulk. Heck, it wouldn't hurt to insist that your guy give you a pre-penetration orgasm via tongue, finger, or toy every time. Just tell him you *couldn't possibly* handle his huge package without one. Buttering him up is the best way to get him to butter *you* up.

MR. HAPPY

(5 to 6 inches [12.7 to 15.2 centimeters] in length and 4 to 5 inches [10.2 to 12.7 centimeters] in circumference)

Most women are more than happy to have a Mr. Happy to play with, as they are perfectly designed to fit snugly within the dimensions of the average woman's vagina. Typically, sexual encounters with these perfectly medium-sized guys leave little to worry about when it comes to trying a variety of sexual positions, because most of them will be a sure fit.

Perfect Positions

Any position is usually a good position with Mr. Happy, but here are a few fun ones you might not have tried before: If you've both been working on your triceps at the gym, try the **Armchair** position. Your guy sits beneath you on a flat surface with his legs extended while supporting his weight on his arms. You sit in his lap facing him and prop your legs up on his shoulders, leaning back, and supporting yourself by your arms. The motion comes from you using your arms to rock back and forth along his cock. This position provides a nice angle for hitting your G-spot.

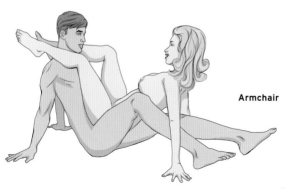

Armchair

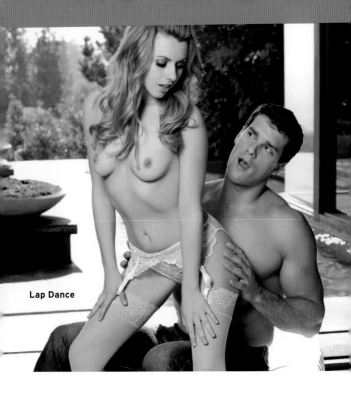

Lap Dance

For a less strenuous but just as sexy position, try the **Lap Dance.** Your man sits on a couch or chair, and you sit in his lap, facing away from him. Grind your way to a delightful climax.

Tasty Tips

One of the best things about Mr. Happy is that his average size makes him perfect for trying some extra-kinky moves and positions—one of our favorites being **Double Penetration.** Add a small- to medium-sized dildo to your sex play and try using it in your anus while Mr. Happy makes your pussy happy (or vice versa). This is a fun way to fulfill your fantasy of a threesome, without the potential jealousy headache. If you find that you like the sensation, be sure to invest in plenty of lube.

THE MAVERICK

(Less than 5 inches [12.7 centimeters] in length and 3.5 inches [8.9 centimeters] or less in circumference)

We call this cock Maverick because it's short and slender, à la Tom Cruise's sexy fighter pilot character in *Top Gun*. There is something quite delightful about finding this loveable lollipop in your guy's underpants. Sure, Maverick may not provide that stretched-to-the-brim feeling that some women love, but sex is about so *much more* than just feeling filled, and that's often where Maverick comes into play. As far as pleasure and true stimulation goes for women, it's only the first 3 inches (7.6 centimeters) of our vaginas that are sensitive to touch—anything deeper and all we feel is pressure. For tickling, teasing, and stroking these sensitive few inches, including the G-spot, Maverick is more than equipped to "buzz the tower" and bring you home to a landing pad of orgasms.

Perfect Positions

Doggy Style is the classic go-to position for mutual enjoyment with Maverick. The trick is positioning: Instead of resting on all fours, lower your arms and head to the bed, so that your ass is sticking up in the air. Arch your spine and draw your thighs together. When he goes in from behind at this angle, Maverick can feel quite large, and this is hands down one of the best positions for hitting your G-spot. As an added bonus, Maverick is one partner with whom Doggy Style will be pain-free—unless, of course, you beg for plenty of spankings to go along with the penetration.

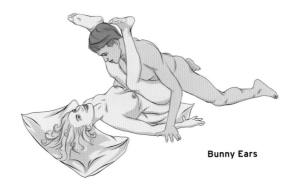

Bunny Ears

Bunny Ears is another position that's just perfect for your Maverick. Lie down on your back, spread your legs, and draw your knees up close to your ears. Have your lover place a pillow under your bottom, and he can also help hold your legs in position. Your pelvis will be tipped in such a way that it will feel like his cock is filling your entire pussy. And, interestingly, this is another great position for prime G-spot stimulation.

Don't overlook the potential pleasure of anal play. Maverick may be just the perfect toy to put in your pretty puckerhole; no pain, just fun. Of course, because Mother Nature didn't equip your booty with its own natural secretions, don't forget to add water-based lube! And last, Maverick may be one of the best penis sizes out there when it comes to giving head. You can suck, lick, tongue, and swallow to your heart's content without ever experiencing the discomfort of gagging or an assault on the back of your throat.

Tasty Tips
If you've already experienced a number of orgasms or heightened arousal beforehand, just the sensation of his hard penis brushing up against your sensitive clit and labia may be enough to send you over

the edge. A man who owns a Maverick is usually an amazing lover because he masters how to pleasure a woman with more than just his cock. But if your Maverick hasn't aced his flight tests yet, why not play sexy flight instructor to this passionate, bad-boy pilot?

To give Maverick a temporary boost in the size department, try having him wear a cock ring (see chapter eight), which can slightly amplify the size of his erection. Also, there is nothing better than incorporating your favorite vibrator into sex play.

THE ACROBAT

(A penis of any size that is bent at a significant angle—either right, left, up, or down)

The challenge with the Acrobat is finding a position that allows for comfortable entry. Happily, you might find that his particular angle can rub you in exactly the right way. (Note that if his bend is very extreme, it could be an indication that he has a medical condition called Peyronie's disease; see chapter eight for more information.)

Perfect Positions

Typically, you are going to want to position your body so that it complements his angle of entry. For example, a guy whose penis curves toward the floor may have better luck entering you from a rear-entry position, such as the **Ben Dover**. Start by standing, and then bend over so that your hands touch the floor with your

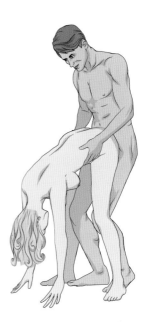

Ben Dover

butt pointed skyward. Your guy then penetrates you comfortably from behind. Note that if he's not much taller than you are, a kneeling Doggy Style position may work better.

Guys with a lefty bend may want to try **Spoons,** a position where you both lie on your right sides and he penetrates you from behind; for the guy with a righty bend, just flip it around and lie on your left sides.

A man whose penis curves up and points back toward his belly button may be able to find his path to paradise with you on top—and lucky for you this is often the best-shaped cock for rubbing your G-spot just right. Try the **Dirty Secretary:** Have him sit upright in an office chair and then straddle him, keeping your feet on the ground for the ultimate in thrusting control.

Tasty Tips

Just because you find one position that works best doesn't mean that you shouldn't explore other options. You'll find the more you explore, the more positions you'll discover that will allow his specially curved penis to rub you in just the right way. The great thing about sex is that, when approached with a smile, it's the trials and errors as well as the orgasmic successes that make it fun!

Remember, ladies, dicks come in a variety of shapes and sizes. We encourage you to get to know the unique plaything that he has hiding in his boxers and make the most of it! Take your time and have fun examining and exploring the many ways his unique penis proportions can pleasure you. This is all an important part of becoming a true penis genius.

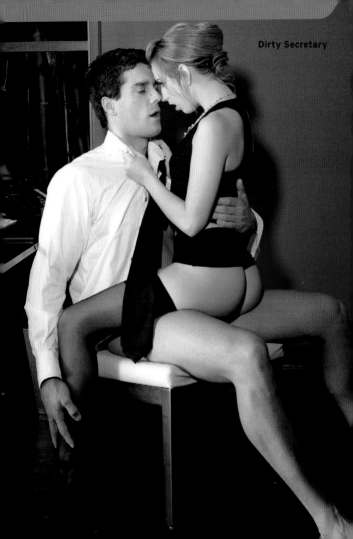

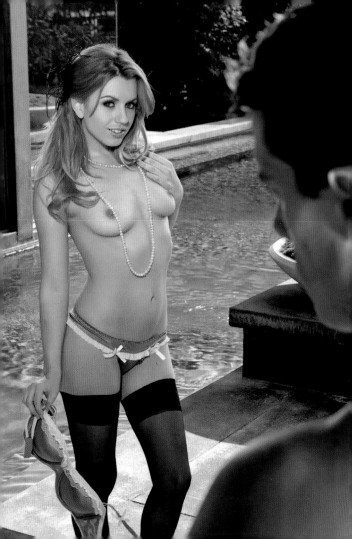

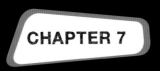

CHAPTER 7

THE PENIS SHRINK: WHAT MAKES HIS OTHER HEAD TICK?

What makes that little head tick? In this chapter, we'll explore different ways his brain and other senses affect the function of his cock. We'll also touch on some of the weirder and funnier manifestations of the human psyche as it relates to the penis.

It's taken for granted that men are visual creatures, and it could be argued that there is a direct connection between his eyes and his cock. Research scientists agree that men experience visual stimuli differently than women. Researchers have found that the amygdala (which is linked to emotions, aggression, and sexual arousal) and hypothalamus (responsible for regulating metabolic processes, among other things) are more strongly activated in men than in women when viewing identical sexual stimuli.

Why not use his sense of sight to your advantage? Knowing that you are visually stimulating your partner can be an incredible turn-on for you as well. Following are some sexy ideas.

DO IT WITH THE LIGHTS ON

Yup, it's that simple! In our survey, we found that 82.5 percent of men prefer sex with the lights on, and 79 percent say they get off more easily when they can see what's happening. This doesn't mean that you have to set up hot stage lights in your bedroom (unless you want to put on a homemade porn production . . . which could be fun). Lord knows that sometimes having the lights turned up makes us a bit self-conscious about whatever we imagine we have to be worried about. (Really, a little cellulite won't send your husband running for the hills, we swear!) There are ways to use your man's wish to see you in the light to get you both in the mood, without lighting up your perceived flaws in the process. Here are a few sexy ways to turn the lights (and him) on:

❶ Early morning light is soft and sexy. Before the sun has risen all the way, open the curtains and let the soft light enhance your lovemaking. Not into first-thing-in-the-morning sex? Get up half an hour early, pee, and brush your teeth, and maybe enjoy a cup of coffee first.

❷ Holiday lights work their magic all year long. Try stringing up a set of white holiday lights around your bedroom, your living room, or even your back patio, wherever you want to feel seductive. Says thirtysomething Phil, "I love to watch my penis enter her—the combination of the sensation of pushing into her and the visual of watching it happen is absolutely incredible! I also love to watch her facial expressions and body's reaction as she builds towards orgasm."

❸ Use a few flickering candles to set the mood. After a romantic meal at home, set the evening on fire with a blazing candelabra and a little sexy lovemaking on the dining room table for dessert. Just don't knock the candles over—even though firemen are sexy, a burning dining room set will ruin the mood.

❹ Lay out a blanket in front of your lit fireplace. The crackling wood, dancing light, and warmth will generate hot passion. Says fortysomething Jeremy, "The shadows of light reflecting off her breasts and outlining her curves are incredibly sensuous! She is a visual delight!"

❺ Use nightlights, ambient light, or a dimly lit doorway for a small amount of light (without the pressure of full-on, 100-watt light bulbs).

Play Dress Up

Men love lingerie. Matching sets of lace undergarments, negligees, and corsets with garters and high-heeled shoes are a few of the fun items you can wear. Don't worry if your expensive silk and lace ends up on the floor more quickly than you had anticipated. That doesn't mean that the lingerie didn't work. Your body in seductive garments simply makes him want to see you entirely naked all the more quickly.

Remember that you don't have to save your lingerie for the bedroom; you can wear it around the house on a lazy Sunday afternoon or wear it while you cook a romantic dinner.

Also note that you don't have to take out stock in Victoria's Secret to get the desired effect. Wear your man's T-shirt with nothing underneath, or try a pair of his underwear with nothing on top.

Looking for a way to showcase all your sexiness? Try putting on a fashion show with your favorite lingerie, heels, or creative outfits of your own making. A scarf tied tightly across your breasts topped by a long jacket provides an alluring silhouette for him to admire!

The Art of Tasteful Flashing

Add a little danger and intrigue to your sex life by carefully flashing your man in unexpected places. The trick is to make sure he is the only one who sees your delectable parts. To make it easy, wear a skirt with nothing underneath. Try discreetly spreading your legs as you take your seat across from him at a dinner party, or briefly flip up the back of your skirt as he trails behind you at the market. Once he realizes you're wearing no panties, he'll lose his mind. Says Charles, a fortysomething attorney, "The sexiest thing my wife does is surprise me by showing me her pussy in a public place."

Have Sex in Front of a Mirror

Double your pleasure by allowing him to enjoy your mirror image while in the throes of passion. Says thirty-seven-year-old Carl, "We have had the opportunity a couple of times to have intercourse in front of a mirror or reflecting window, and we both enjoy watching our bodies' reactions, the penetration, and the fucking." Bend over the bathroom sink so he can get a nice image of your face and breasts in the mirror while he simultaneously enjoys the view of your backside. Mirrored headboards, ceilings, and closet doors can also offer a delightful visual treat. For a super-dirty twist, when you're on all fours in Doggy Style, use a hand mirror to show him the view from beneath your body.

Masturbate for Him

When we asked our men what the sexiest thing a woman has ever done to visually stimulate them, far and away the most common response was that their lovers masturbated for them. If you feel shy, get yourself in the mood by warming up before the show. Here are some ideas:

❶ Start masturbating before he comes in the room and let him "catch you" in the act.

❷ Ask him to give you a little oral sex first to get you in the proper state of mind.

❸ Wear a blindfold so you can completely close him out and just allow yourself to let go.

❹ Watch him masturbate for you while you play with yourself for him.

❺ Don't be afraid to add your favorite sex toy. Says fiftysomething Christopher, "The sexiest thing my wife ever did for me was let me watch as she masturbated with her dildo."

Anything that will bring you to orgasm will make the experience that much more exciting . . . for the both of you!

Sexy Photos and Films

Titillate your man by taking sexy photos of yourself or filming the two of you together so you can watch later. Your man will appreciate being able to relive your sexiness when you're not around. Moreover, the act of taking photos or videos during sex adds elements of exhibitionism and voyeurism that can be incredibly arousing for both parties. Says twentysomething Ray, "The sexiest thing my girlfriend does for me is to send erotic videos to my phone when I'm least expecting it."

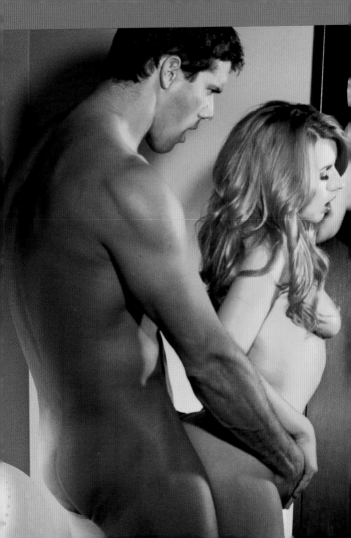

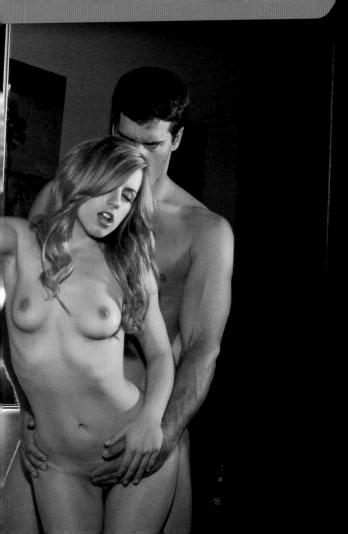

A word of warning: Be aware in this day and age of the rapid sharing of information. It's best if you only share photos with someone who you completely trust and remove any identifying features from anything you send over the Internet or by cell phone. And if you are a high-profile politician who could risk losing your career, it's probably best to not partake in this type of activity at all.

STRESSED OUT!

Stress can be a big factor in your guy's brain-to-penis connection. Of the men we surveyed, 60 percent reported that stress negatively affects their desire for sex. "When stressed, I can't even think about sex," says fortysomething Arnold.

Dr. Maryrose Gerardi of Emory University explains that the reason stress can cause a decrease in desire is simply because of fatigue. People who work over forty-eight hours per week or who don't get enough sleep often will lose their sex drive.

Tips for Destressing Your Man

If your man's flagpole is at half-mast thanks to stress, here are some ideas to help him slow down and reconnect:

❶ Give him an erotic massage. Not only are massages inherently relaxing, but they are sensual and can lead to sex. (For tips on giving a massage, read chapter four).

❷ Have a sexy Sunday. Encourage him to sleep in, fix him breakfast in bed, and relax with a movie marathon interspersed with blow jobs, sex, and lots of snuggles.

❸ Take a vacation. Even if it's just for a weekend, a change of scenery can do wonders for stress levels. Don't forget to pack a bag full of lingerie and sex toys.

On the flip side, sex can be a great way to relieve stress, and sometimes people turn to sex as a release when everything around them seems to be falling apart. In fact, 34 percent of the men we surveyed say that sometimes stress has the opposite effect and makes them want more sex. Trey, a fortysomething health regulator, says, "When I'm under pressure at work, it makes me horny and therefore sex is more intense and enjoyable." If you have one of these stress-loving studs, more power to you!

CHEATING BASTARDS

According to the University of Chicago's General Social Survey (GSS) that spanned the course of eleven years, researchers found that men are about twice as likely as women to cheat on their spouses. Five percent of men and 2.5 percent of women reported infidelity during a twelve-month time frame with their current spouse. Twenty-two percent of men and 12 percent of women reported having ever cheated in their lives.

While our survey sample size was smaller and included nonmarried men, 43 percent of them admitted to having cheated. What's more, 76 percent of these guys said that cheating did *not* affect their ability to perform with their primary partners.

Renowned biological anthropologist Dr. Helen Fisher explains why some people are able to cheat: "We've evolved three distinct brain systems for mating and reproduction. One is a sex drive, one is romantic love, and the third brain system is for attachment. . . . And these three brain systems aren't always well connected. You can feel deep attachment for one person, while you feel intense romantic love for someone else, while you feel the sex drive for a host of other individuals . . . the brain is built to enable us to love more than one person at a time. This is not to say that biology is destiny; we have an enormous cerebral cortex with which we make decisions . . . you can say no to adultery."

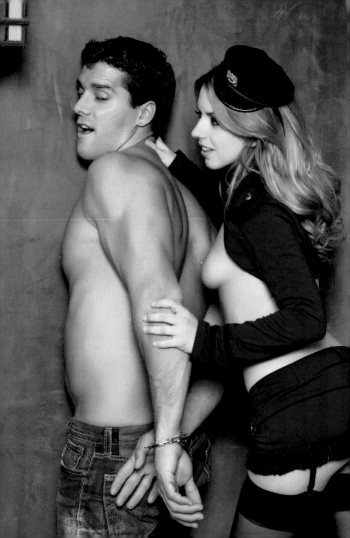

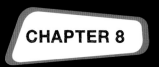

CHAPTER 8

DISORDERLY CONDUCT: DIFFICULT PROBLEMS THAT CAN POP UP

His dick is subject to a variety of disorders, both physical and psychosomatic, from ejaculation and erection difficulties to pains in the penis and sexually transmitted infections. In this chapter, we'll discuss some of the problems that can pop up and tell you how to successfully sexually navigate your way through them for a healthier Mr. Happy.

ERECTILE DYSFUNCTION

Erectile dysfunction (ED) is basically a fancy way of saying that he can't get it up. A temporary mechanical failure can happen to any guy—particularly in the case of whiskey dick, a condition resulting from consuming too much alcohol. Other times, the malfunction doesn't have as ready an explanation. However, some men have erection problems more frequently and for more serious reasons, which can wreak havoc on their sex lives and their confidence.

The causes of ED fall into two broad categories: physical and psychological. Does your guy get boners while he sleeps? If he is still constructing morning wood, his ED is all in his head. However, if his prick is floppy morning, noon, and night, he may have a physical condition that is blocking blood flow to his boner.

Physical Problems That Can Cause a Droopy Member

Diabetes, high blood pressure, obesity, vascular disease, surgery, side effects from smoking, drinking, drugs (prescribed or otherwise), and a host of other physical causes can disrupt an erection. Some of these problems are easily solved, such as taking medications to lower high blood pressure. But other problems may be more complex, such as in some cases of diabetes. Diabetes can damage the blood vessels and nerves that control erections.

Psychological Problems That Can Cause a Misbehaving Hard-on

Relationship stress such as cheating partners, financial troubles, or frequent arguing over who gets to wake up at 3 a.m. to change poopy diapers can all impede a boner. He may also have hang-ups left over from his religious upbringing (no one wants to go to hell for ejaculating), or from sexual abuse that occurred in his childhood.

The most common psychological problem is performance anxiety. This is a temporary manifestation of ED that results when a guy psychs himself out before the big (bedroom) game. If, for example, the first time he tries to please you in the sack his penis fails him, subsequent attempts may be foiled by his belief that he won't be able to get it up . . . ever again. Performance anxiety is the easiest issue to address, because all it takes is a little patience and encouragement to get him back into tip-top fucking condition. Says Jay, a fiftysomething technician, "ED happened to me only once. Funny thing is, I think it was because she was so excited to finally get to be with me and she kept telling me so, which made me feel pressured. She didn't get too upset with me when my erection failed, so everything ended up fine and the next morning we got to it."

Tips for Expertly Handling a Dysfunctional Erection

❶ **Don't blame yourself!** You might feel like you are somehow failing your man because you are unable to help him achieve an erection. Avoid the desire to ask him what you did wrong, and try not to overanalyze or pick apart the situation. It's best to let it slide, so he isn't stressed out about his erection the next time he has a chance to play.

❷ **Be compassionate**. Men put a lot of stock in their ability to perform sexually. Don't poke fun at his suffering; this will only exacerbate the problem.

❸ **Think outside the cock**. Sometimes the best sex is had without the usual penis-plunging-into-vagina action. This is a great opportunity to employ tongue, fingers, and toys to achieve amazing and long-lasting pleasure. You may find that you'll enjoy more and better orgasms.

❹ **Treasure his pleasure map**. Your man can be sexually stimulated even with a slumbering penis. Massages, nibbling, tickling, and teasing him all over can bring him great pleasure. And who knows, he may even surprise you both by rising to the occasion!

❺ Consult an M.D. If the problem is physical, your man should consult his doctor to see if the underlying health issue can be resolved. Sometimes, all it takes is quitting smoking or beginning an exercise routine and eating more vegetables to get everything back in working order. If the problem is disease related, a physician may be able to assist by prescribing an ED medication.

❻ Consult a Ph.D. If the issue is psychological, usually patience, kindness, and time will work wonders to solve his mental hang-ups. But if he needs more help, your man should consult a licensed sex therapist who can work with him to uncover any underlying issues.

DELAYED EJACULATION

Delayed ejaculation refers to when a man requires extra-long lovin' to ejaculate (thirty minutes or more). It can also describe a condition in which he can't ejaculate at all, no matter how much stimulation he receives. Delayed ejaculation is only a problem if it negatively interferes with your sex life. Sometimes, the issue can be permanent, while other times it's only temporary, and, like ED, it can be caused by either physical or psychological issues. Lawrence, a twenty-nine-year-old playwright, says, "I suffered from delayed ejaculation. Often, I would stay hard for a very long time without being able to come. This was [based on] a psychological fear of getting a girl pregnant. I have overcome it somewhat, but it still takes me a while."

Antidepressants and high blood pressure medications, as well as marijuana and alcohol abuse, can cause delayed ejaculation. Other physical causes include birth defects, spinal cord injury, surgery, prostate or urinary tract infections, and diabetes. Delayed ejaculation should not be confused with retrograde ejaculation, which is when your guy orgasms but doesn't spurt. In cases of retrograde ejaculation, his semen has gone the wrong way down the sperm highway and exited into his bladder.

Tips for Handling Your "Love You Long Time" Lover

❶ **Enjoy it**. If your guy's delayed ejaculation is not a symptom of a larger health concern, take advantage of his endurance sex. You may find that his sexual response cycle is more in line with your own and that he'll last long enough to allow you to achieve your sought-after orgasm. (Or if you're even luckier—multiple orgasms!)

❷ **Warm him up**. If your pussy gets tired after, say, more than 100 thrusts, get him started long before penetration. Have him masturbate for you, give him a warm-up blow job, or use a sex toy (such as a masturbation sleeve) on him to get things heated up. When he's obviously getting closer to ejaculation, you can send in your home-run hitter.

❸ **Lay off the booze and drugs**. If your guy is a heavy drinker or drug user, adopting a healthier lifestyle can bring him that much closer to being able to achieve his goals.

❹ **See an M.D.** If you suspect his problem is related to prescription medications or an underlying health issue, see a doctor.

❺ **See a Ph.D.** If your guy can't come due to debilitating psychological issues stemming from childhood sexual abuse, religious indoctrination, depression, or relationship stresses, he should see a sex therapist to overcome these hurdles.

PREMATURE EJACULATION

Premature ejaculation (PE) describes the sexual situation in which your guy ejaculates sooner than he would like to. This becomes problematic when his hasty hard-on consistently makes it to the big-O finish line before you do. Any committed girl who has to rely solely on BOB (battery-operated boyfriend) to achieve all of her orgasms knows that PE can become a bit exasperating. Lucky for you and your little friend, the problem is usually an easy fix and you might be able to leave BOB in the drawer next time you do the mattress mambo.

Tips for Handling Your "Quick Draw McGraw"

❶ **Play red light, green light**. The easiest, most natural, and effective way to combat PE is known as the start-stop method. First, your guy needs to rate his arousal on a scale of 1 to 10, 1 being getting a cavity filled and 10 being spurting cum all over your breasts. During a sexual encounter, have your guy bring himself to about level 7, but before he pushes any further he must stop everything (red light!) until he relaxes back to a level 3 or 4, at which point he can rev his engines back up (green light!). Have him repeat this sequence three full times before allowing orgasm. Start by using your hands and lube, and eventually try it inside the overwhelmingly arousing confines of your body. Be patient and allow him plenty of practice. Over time, your guy will learn how to extend his performance and ejaculate at will—a boon for the both of you!

❷ **Foreplay.** It's common for women to take longer to achieve orgasm than men. For a woman who is dating a man with a much shorter arousal cycle than her own, foreplay is the best way to obtain mutual satisfaction. Make it a household rule that you always come first and encourage your three-pump chump to bring you to your big O before he gets invited inside to play. Most women find satisfaction in oral or finger play before penetration. To add more excitement, reveal your secret dildo and let him do the dirty work while you lie back and enjoy the sensations. Only when he's successfully driven you over the crest of orgasm hill can he climb on for his own ride.

❸ Extending creams. There are a variety of desensitizing creams available at sex toy stores. These creams usually use benzocaine, which is a numbing agent. The idea is to desensitize him to the pleasures of your pussy so that it will take him longer to come. Before you buy, do your research and read reviews by other users. Some creams have a bitter flavor, which means you won't be able to give him a blow job, while others are so strong that they'll have the unfortunate side effect of numbing you in the process (using a condom will help with this issue), and other creams just don't work at all.

❹ Cock rings. Wrap one of these little devices around the base of your man's prick to trap blood in his penis, allowing for bigger and longer-lasting erections.

SEXUALLY TRANSMITTED INFECTIONS

Because sex is a human-to-human interaction that involves the exchange of a veritable cocktail of bodily fluids (more than you'd ever exchange by sharing a carton of milk), the risk of sexually transmitted infections (STIs) should be taken seriously. Before toying with your boy toy, you'll want to find out if your partner is drug and disease free. (Sometimes, this isn't possible, especially if you are jumping into bed with that hotty you met in the produce section. It's not typical to discuss sexual histories while flirting over ripe fruit.) Ultimately, the best way to prevent STIs is to be in a committed monogamous relationship, but if that isn't preferable to you, use condoms every single time.

Chlamydia

Chlamydia shows its ugly face on the penis by way of inflammation of the urinary tract, causing painful peeing or a discharge of pus or mucus from the meatus. Symptoms usually occur within three weeks of exposure. Treatment for chlamydia is simple and consists of a short series of antibiotics. If untreated, your guy's nuts may swell up like balloons, and he could develop a painful reactive arthritis called

Reiter syndrome, which is a real pain in the penis and can cause lesions, incontinence, and other unsavory issues.

Gonorrhea

Gonorrhea is chlamydia's ugly sister and shows up in the form of a white or yellowish discharge from the penis accompanied by a painful burning sensation while urinating. Your guy can also get the gunk in his rectum, causing an itching butthole and painful poops. Symptoms usually occur within ten days of exposure. Usually, gonorrhea is treated at the same time as chlamydia with a simple series of antibiotics.

Human Papillomavirus

Human papillomavirus, or HPV, is one of the most common STIs, and it comes in at least sixty different viral flavors. The Center for Disease Control (CDC) reports that at least 50 percent of sexually active people will get some form of HPV in their lives. Some varieties of HPV can cause penile cancer, which is rare. Unfortunately, it isn't easy to spot a prick with HPV, because it's uncommon for a man to manifest any symptoms. Only a few strains of the virus show up as occasional outbreaks of genital warts. Moreover, women are susceptible to developing cervical cancer as a result of the virus.

The CDC recommends that men aged twenty-six or younger receive the Gardasil vaccine, which will protect them from most strains of HPV that cause genital warts. Condoms may lower the risk of HPV, but because the virus is transmitted from skin-to-skin contact, condoms won't cover the entire affected area (such as the pubic region and testicles), and aren't 100 percent effective.

Genital Herpes

Herpes infect about 16 percent of Americans between fourteen and forty-nine years old, including one out of nine men. It's more likely for a man to give a woman this unwanted gift than the other way around. Herpes show up as blistering sores on the genitals that last from several days to several weeks, and will pop up randomly as long as a person is carrying the virus (which typically lasts a lifetime).

Between outbreaks, it will appear to be all systems normal. However, these tricky buggers can be transmitted even when there are no sores. It's best to use condoms at all times, which can reduce the risk of sharing this fun little virus. The use of antiviral medications can help prevent outbreaks, and some people with frequent outbreaks (six or more times per year) can be put on daily suppressive therapy (a daily dose of antiviral meds such as Valtrex) to prevent sores from rearing their icky lil' heads.

Syphilis

Syphilis has plagued civilization since the sixteenth century. Before the days of penicillin, it could not be treated and caused the suffering and death of many. Today, the syphilis bacteria still infect people, but is usually discovered and treated early with a dose of antibiotics. There are four stages of this nasty disease. In the first stage, a single, small chancre sore develops on the genitals. In the second stage, the chancre will disappear and be replaced by a rash of rough red spots on the hands and feet, sometimes accompanied by flu-like symptoms, weight loss, and hair loss. In the third stage, the rash and symptoms will disappear and the syphilis will stay latent in the body for up to twenty years before attacking the organs, including the brain, liver, eyes, bones, and more. The last stage can cause paralysis, numbness, dementia, blindness, and death. Prevent this from happening to you (and your lovers) by using condoms and regularly getting tested for syphilis along with other STIs.

Crabs (Pubic Lice)

Unlike many other STIs, the symptoms are obvious throughout the infection. They cause itching and, if looked at closely, you can see them with the naked eye. Crabs cozy up in the coarse pubic hair in the form of eggs, which eventually hatch and grow into adults. They can't survive outside the moist, warm environment of the human body. To get rid of these disgusting creatures, try over-the-counter lice-killing lotions. If this doesn't work, visit your doctor for a prescription-strength solution.

HIV/AIDS

HIV/AIDS is the most pernicious STI of our time. HIV is a human immunodeficiency virus that leads to AIDS (acquired immunodeficiency syndrome). The first known case of the infection was detected in a blood sample taken from a man in the Democratic Republic of the Congo in 1959. Researchers believe the virus originated in chimpanzees in West Africa and was introduced to human hunters who came in contact with their blood. The disease became a full-blown epidemic in the United States in the 1980s.

HIV attacks the immune system and can cause rapid deterioration in health by making sufferers more susceptible to diseases such as pneumonia and cancers that cause death. HIV/AIDS is transmitted by direct exposure to blood and semen and is thus most commonly transmitted via unprotected sex and intravenous drug use with shared needles. Unlike STIs that are transmitted from skin-to-skin contact, the virus is highly preventable during sex by using condoms. More than twenty years of medical research and progress have produced drugs that actively and effectively suppress the virus and allow people to live fairly normal lives. Also, a drug cocktail known as antiretroviral therapy, or ART, has been shown to decrease the risk of HIV transmission. However, this STI stands alone as reason enough to always practice safer sex.

PENIS-SPECIFIC PROBLEMS

Since these odd little issues can surface on any penis, it's a good idea to learn how to recognize them and know what to do about them.

Peyronie's Disease

If you notice your man's penis bending at an extreme angle and sex has become painful for him, he may have Peyronie's disease. The condition is caused by a series of microfractures or traumas (e.g., getting hit in the crotch with a baseball, or bending his penis in a sloppy attempt to copulate) that lead to calcification, scarring, and deformation of the penis. In some cases, the issue will resolve itself over time. Other cases may be treated with prescribed oral medicines and injections, and severe cases may require surgery.

Priapism

Priapism is a painful erection that develops for nonsexual reasons and won't go away. Physiologically, blood becomes trapped in the penis. Priapism is often caused by ED medications gone haywire. Other causes include sickle-cell anemia, genital trauma, black widow spider bites, and cocaine and marijuana use. To treat the problem, apply ice packs to his genitals. If this doesn't make the erection subside, your guy will have to head to the emergency room, where they may have to aspirate his penis by inserting a needle and draining blood from his boner. In some extreme cases, his penis may be injected with a drug that causes his veins to narrow and reduce blood flow, or surgical intervention may be required.

Balanitis

Balanitis is an inflammation of the skin of his glans and is more common among uncircumcised males with poor hygiene. The condition can be brought about by a buildup of smegma under the foreskin, which, in turn, causes a stinky, itchy, inflamed rash. Balanitis can also be caused by diabetes, obesity, penile cancer, an allergy to soaps, spermicides or other products, a yeast infection, or it can be the result of an STI. If your man develops this condition, he should seek medical attention immediately so that the underlying cause can be determined and he can be treated appropriately by a physician.

While we like to think that sex is always fun and carefree, it's good to remember that sometimes problems can pop up. The best way to equip yourself to handle these sticky or icky situations is to educate yourself, take precautions, and act when necessary.

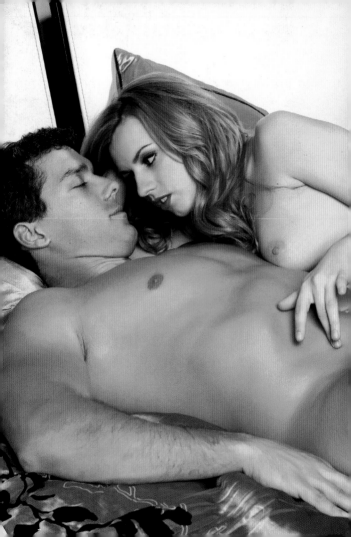

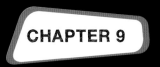

CHAPTER 9

A HAPPY, HEALTHY PENIS: PROTECTING YOUR (AND HIS) FAVORITE PLAYTHING FOR A LIFETIME

Just as he takes extra-special care of his sports car, motorcycle, or boat, your guy should take care of his penis as if it were a valuable possession. After all, a sexy sex life is an important component to a happy life, and the health of his cock is linked to his overall health. Let's talk about the best ways to take care of your (and his) favorite plaything for life.

KEGEL EXERCISES: WHAT ARE THEY GOOD FOR?

Kegel exercises were initially developed by the gynecologist Dr. Arnold Kegel to help treat women who developed urinary incontinence after childbirth. However, the technique isn't only beneficial to women. It's also been found to help men keep their prostates healthy, avoid incontinence, increase sexual pleasure, and even treat premature ejaculation.

Kegel exercises are performed by squeezing the pubococcygeus (PC) muscle of the pelvic floor. The PC muscle cradles the pelvic area in both men and women, running from the pubic bone to the tailbone. When he squeezes his PC muscle, he may feel a lift to his testicles and a tightening of the anal sphincter muscle. Performed daily, Kegels will improve the long-term health of his private parts.

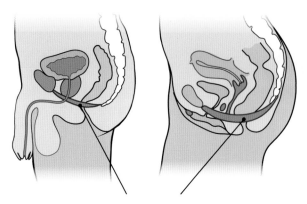

PC muscles in a man and woman

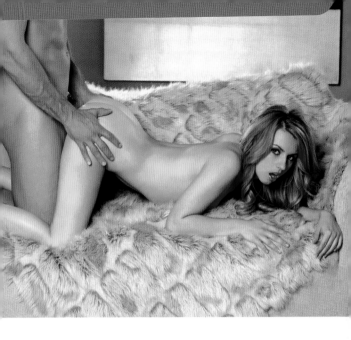

EJACULATION IS GOOD FOR HIM

Scientists agree: Ejaculation is good for your man, and because it doesn't carry the same risks of acquiring sexually transmitted infections, ejaculation via masturbation is even better.

In a 2004 study carried out by the National Cancer Institute, 342 men were evaluated over the course of eight years, during which time frequency of ejaculation was compared with the development of prostate cancer. The study found that "high ejaculation frequency was related to *decreased* risk of total prostate cancer." Men who masturbated twenty-one or more times per month fared better than those who ejaculated four to seven times per month.

This study is backed up by another conducted in 2003 by Graham Giles of the Cancer Council Australia. The researchers found that men who ejaculated five times or more per week in their twenties were one-third less likely to develop prostate cancer later. In an interview with *New Scientist*, Giles attributed his findings to what he calls the "prostatic stagnation hypothesis," which basically proposes that men who ejaculate frequently cleanse their prostates and help prevent the buildup of carcinogens. Perhaps there is a shadow of truth, then, behind the urban myth DSB (deadly sperm backup). DSB is the male equivalent of PMS and is said to occur when a man isn't getting laid enough, which causes moodiness and sometimes death. Next time your man is whining over the remote and cracking open your chocolate almond fudge ice cream, lovingly remind him that it may be time for him to "crack one off" instead.

Tips on Healthy Ejaculation

How frequently a man can ejaculate depends on multiple factors, including his overall health, his age, and his unique sex drive. Here are some ways you can make sure he's keeping his prostate clear and ready for takeoff:

❶ **Learn how to give a prostate massage.** If what scientists are saying is true, giving prostate massages can keep the fluids flowing and help prevent bad stuff from backing up in his pipes. (Read chapter four for more information on how to give a prostate massage.)

❷ **Participate in the fun**. With his sexy scientist around, your man doesn't have to always go it alone. Masturbate with him and add a little excitement to your sexual repertoire. Pick out a porn movie together, or order a set of his and hers sex toys and enjoy the fun of mutual masturbation. You can either masturbate each other, or enjoy your own private voyeur/exhibitionist game.

❸ **Sex is good for you**. Make it a goal to increase the number of times you and your partner have sex. If you partner up once a month, try going for it once per week. If you have a once-weekly ritual, up the ante to three or four times per week. If you are already going at it like bunnies, kudos to you! You'll find that the more sex you have, the more you'll both want.

A happy penis brings with it the benefits of better overall health and a more satisfying sex life. Keep your plaything in top condition by practicing Kegels, observing a healthy and active lifestyle, and enjoying frequent sex, and you'll both reap great rewards in and out of the bedroom.

ABOUT THE AUTHORS

Jordan LaRousse and **Samantha Sade** are co-owners and co-editors of *Oysters & Chocolate* (www.oystersandchocolate.com), an online magazine for women's erotica. The site is home to hundreds of erotic stories and poems, sex-advice Q&A column "Ask Jordan," and numerous erotic toy, video, website, and product reviews. The duo strives to not only provide quality literary erotica, but to engage women from all walks of life in the topic of sex in a fun and informative way.